4e

MOSBY'S

RN

Nursing Facts at Hand

practical • detailed • quick

Consultant
Rae W. Langford, EdD, RN, MS

ELSEVIER

ELSEVIER

3251 Riverport Lane
St. Louis, Missouri 63043

MOSBY'S PDQ FOR RN, FOURTH EDITION
ISBN: 978-0-323-40028-2
Copyright © 2017 by Elsevier, Inc. All rights reserved.

Notices

Knowledge and best practice in this field are constantly changing. As new research and experience broaden our understanding, changes in research methods, professional practices, or medical treatment may become necessary.

Practitioners and researchers must always rely on their own experience and knowledge in evaluating and using any information, methods, compounds, or experiments described herein. In using such information or methods they should be mindful of their own safety and the safety of others, including parties for whom they have a professional responsibility.

With respect to any drug or pharmaceutical products identified, readers are advised to check the most current information provided (i) on procedures featured or (ii) by the manufacturer of each product to be administered, to verify the recommended dose or formula, the method and duration of administration, and contraindications. It is the responsibility of practitioners, relying on their own experience and knowledge of their patients, to make diagnoses, to determine dosages and the best treatment for each individual patient, and to take all appropriate safety precautions.

To the fullest extent of the law, neither the Publisher nor the authors, contributors, or editors, assume any liability for any injury and/or damage to persons or property as a matter of products liability, negligence or otherwise, or from any use or operation of any methods, products, instructions, or ideas contained in the material herein.

Previous editions copyrighted 2013, 2008, and 2004.

LCCN 2015032026

Content Strategist: Kristin Geen
Content Development Manager: Billie C. Sharp
Content Development Specialist: Samantha Dalton
Publishing Services Manager: Jeff Patterson
Project Manager: Lisa A. P. Bushey
Designer: Ashley Miner

Printed in China
Last digit is the print number: 9 8 7 6 5 4

PROCEDURES

SEE ALSO

MEDS/IV

PEDIATRICS

PROCEDURES

This section describes a variety of nursing procedures. Although not specifically stated, it is expected that the nurse will check physician orders, obtain appropriate equipment, discuss the procedure to be performed with the patient, take appropriate infection control measures (wash hands, wear gloves, etc.), and document each procedure.

INFECTION CONTROL

Standard Precautions[52, 68]

Purpose: Used to prevent hospital acquired infections—applied to all patients.

- **Hand hygiene:** Two acceptable methods for hand hygiene:
  - *Handwashing (HW)* with antiseptic soap and water by rubbing hands together vigorously for 15 seconds covering all surface areas
  - *Decontamination (D)* with alcohol-based hand rub by applying product to palm of one hand and rubbing hands together, covering all surfaces of hands and fingers, until hands are dry

  Indications:
  - Before and after patient contact, even when gloves are worn (D)
  - After contact with objects/equipment in patient environment (D)
  - Hands are visibly dirty or contaminated (HW)
  - Before and after eating (HW)
  - Before/after eating or using toilet (HW)
  - Exposure to spore-forming organisms (HW)
- **Gloves:** Worn whenever contact with body fluids is likely.

- **Mask and/or eye cover:** Worn when splashing of body fluids is likely.
- **Gown:** Worn when soiling of exposed skin or clothing is likely.
- **Needles/sharps:** Do not recap or break needles; discard all sharp objects immediately in a puncture-resistant container.
- Properly clean or discard patient care equipment.
- Place contaminated linen in a leak-proof bag.

Transmission-Based Precautions[51, 56]

CATEGORY	DISEASE	BARRIER PROTECTION
Airborne precautions	Diseases transmitted by small droplet nuclei (smaller than 5 microns), such as measles, chickenpox, TB, etc.	Private room; negative airflow of at least 6-12 air exchanges per hr via HEPA filtration; mask or respirator (N95) required
Droplet precautions	Diseases transmitted by large droplets from mucous membranes, nose, mouth (larger than 5 microns), such as streptococcal pharyngitis, pertussis, mumps, pneumonic plague, meningococcal pneumonia, etc.	Private room; mask or respirator when within 3 feet of patient required depending on condition (refer to agency policy)
Contact precautions	Diseases transmitted by direct patient or environmental contact, such as colonization or infection with drug-resistant organisms, enteric pathogens, wound infections, herpes simplex, scabies, RSV, etc.	Private room; gloves; gown; See agency policy.

Note: For Ebola virus precautions- Access CDC guidelines at www.cdc.gov/vhf/ebola/healthcare-us/hospitals/infection-control.html

▰ SPECIMEN COLLECTION ▰

Nasal/Throat Specimens[52]

Purpose: Obtain nasal or throat specimen for culture.

1. Have patient sit erect in bed and tilt head back.
2. Don gloves; loosen tube top on culture tubes.
3. Collect nasal culture:
   a. Have patient blow nose.
   b. Assess nasal passages for patency (use nasal speculum if needed).
   c. Gently swab any inflamed or purulent areas.
   d. Withdraw swab carefully; avoid touching the nasal speculum.
   e. Place swab into culture tube and crush ampule in bottom of tube to release culture medium.
   f. Ensure that swab tip is immersed in the medium liquid and secure top on the tube.
4. Collect throat culture:
   a. Have patient open throat and say "ah."
   b. Assess throat for inflammation and drainage.
   c. Use tongue depressor to flatten tongue.
   d. Insert swab without touching lips, teeth, tongue, cheeks, or uvula.
   e. Gently and quickly swab tonsillar pillars, making contact with inflamed purulent sites.
   f. Withdraw swab carefully, avoiding all oral structures.
   g. Place swab into culture tube and crush ampule in bottom of tube to release culture medium.
   h. Ensure that swab tip is immersed in the medium liquid and secure top on the tube.

Urine Specimen[52]

Random specimen	• Patient voids in specimen container. Document time, label specimen container, send to laboratory.
Sterile specimen	• Clean catch (female): Instruct patient to clean meatus, void small amount into toilet while separating labia; without interrupting flow, catch urine stream in specimen cup.
	• Clean catch (male): Instruct patient to pull back foreskin, clean meatus, void small amount into toilet; without interrupting flow, catch urine stream in specimen cup.
	• From indwelling catheter: Clamp tubing distal to collection port. After 15-30 minutes, clean collection port with disinfectant and aspirate urine from port using a needleless Luer-Lok syringe; place in clean specimen cup for urinalysis or sterile cup for culture; Unclamp catheter.
	• Document time, label specimen container, send to laboratory.
24-hour urine	• To begin, instruct patient to void and discard urine, record time.
	• For the next 24 hours, collect urine from all subsequent voids and place in a single sealed container—usually container is kept on ice or in refrigerated specimen area.
	• At end of 24-hour period, instruct patient to void and add this final urine specimen to container.
	• Record date and time; label specimen container, send to laboratory.

Venipuncture for Blood Specimen Collection[50]

Purpose: Obtain a venous blood sample for laboratory analysis.

1. Select vein for venipuncture (usually ante-cubital space).*

2. Apply tourniquet 2-4 inches above intended puncture site and palpate vein.

3. Clean venipuncture site (with antiseptic swab); allow area to dry.

4. Perform venipuncture by entering the skin with needle at approximately a 15-degree angle to the skin, needle bevel up.

5. If using a _Vacutainer_, ease tube forward in holder once in the vein. If using a _syringe_, pull back on the barrel with slow, even tension as blood fills the syringe.

6. Release tourniquet when the blood begins to flow.

7. After blood is drawn, place gauze pad over site; withdraw the needle and exert pressure. Apply bandage if needed.

8. Mix additive tubes with gentle rolling motion (do not vigorously shake tubes). If specimens collected in syringe, transfer to appropriate tubes.

9. Properly dispose of contaminated materials.

10. Record the date and time of blood collection. Attach a label to each blood tube.

*_Note: Do not use a vein site proximal to an IV infusion._

Arterial Puncture for Specimen Collection[50]

Purpose: Obtain arterial blood sample for laboratory analysis.

1. Perform Allen test to assess collateral circulation before performing arterial puncture on radial artery. Apply pressure over radial and ulnar arteries to obliterate blood flow; hand should blanch. Release pressure over ulnar artery; a flushing color indicates adequate collateral circulation. Failure to flush is a negative result meaning that radial artery should not be used, and other arm should be tested. If Allen test is negative in both arms, choose alternative site for arterial puncture.

2. Clean site with antiseptic swab; allow to dry.

3. Attach 20-gauge needle to a syringe containing 0.2 mL of heparin; insert needle at 45- to 60-degree angle into skin directly over where artery is palpable.

4. Draw 2-3 mL of blood, remove needle, and apply pressure to puncture site for 3-5 min (15 min if patient is on anticoagulant therapy).

5. Expel air bubbles if present, place cap on syringe, and gently rotate to mix blood and heparin.

6. Place arterial blood on ice and immediately take to laboratory for analysis. On laboratory slip, indicate amount of oxygen administration and/or any mechanical ventilation.

Common Blood Collection Tubes[50]

COLOR TOP	ADDITIVE	PURPOSE	EXAMPLES
Red	None	Allows blood sample to clot. Permits separation of serum when the serum needs to be tested	Chemistry, Bilirubin, Calcium, BUN
Light blue	Sodium citrate	Prevents blood sample from clotting when plasma needs to be tested	Coagulation studies (PT, PTT, etc.)
Green	Heparin	Prevents blood sample from clotting when plasma needs to be tested	Chemistry, Ammonia, Carboxyhemoglobin
Purple or lavender	EDTA	Prevents blood sample from clotting	Hematology, CBC, Platelet Count
Red and black speckled, or gold (serum separator tubes)	Inert silicon gel	Separates red cells and serum after centrifuging	Chemistry, Serology
Gray	Sodium fluoride oxalate	Prevents glycolysis of blood sample	Chemistry, Glucose, Lactose tolerance

CBC, complete blood count; **EDTA**, ethylenediamine tetraacetic acid; **PT**, prothrombin time; **PTT**, partial thromboplastin time.

BLOOD ADMINISTRATION

Administration of a Blood Transfusion[52]

Purpose: IV replacement of blood components.

1. Check patient's baseline data prior to initiating infusion (vital signs and other appropriate laboratory findings).
2. Obtain blood product from blood bank. With another licensed caregiver, verify blood product by checking the following:
   - Patient states first and last name while nurse verifies name on blood bank arm band
   - Correct blood product ordered
   - Blood type and Rh factor of donor blood with patient type and Rh
   - Unit number on blood product matches the arm band and blood bank form
   - Expiration date/time noted on blood bag
3. Document verification process per institution policy.
4. Prepare the blood component.
   - Spike a 0.9% NaCl IV bag with a Y Blood Tubing set. Prime entire blood tubing line and filter, clamp tubing. **(Never use any component fluid other than 0.9% NaCl.)**
   - Insert other spike into blood bag.
5. Infuse blood product (use IV pump if available).
   - Open the roller clamp to blood bag; allow blood to flow at desired rate (slowly for the first 15 min).
   - Monitor vital signs during transfusion according to agency policy.
   - Monitor patient for blood transfusion reactions.
   - Administer most transfusions over about 2 hrs; never exceed 4 hrs.

Types of Blood Products

PRODUCT	ACTION/USES
Whole blood	Replacement of RBCs and plasma volume to raise Hgb and HCT levels. Not commonly used due to problems with fluid overload.
PRBCs	Preferred source for replacement of RBCs to raise Hgb and HCT levels. Contains RBCs without plasma volume. Used to treat severe or symptomatic anemia or acute blood loss.
Fresh frozen plasma	Replacement of plasma without RBCs or platelets. Contains most coagulation factors except platelets. Used to control bleeding caused by deficiency in clotting factors.
Platelets	Replacement of platelets. Used to treat severe or symptomatic thrombocytopenia.
Albumin	A hyperosmolar solution prepared from plasma that expands vascular volume. Used to treat hypovolemic shock or hypoalbuminemia.

HCT, hematocrit; **Hgb**, hemoglobin; **PRBC**, packed red blood cell; **RBC**, red blood cell.

Transfusion Reactions[6, 52]

TRANSFUSION REACTION	SYMPTOMS	TREATMENT
Acute hemolytic reaction Usually occurs within 5-15 min after initiation of transfusion.	• Hypotension • Burning in vein • Flushed face • Headache • Diffuse pain	• Stop transfusion • Start NS or LR • Consider diuretics • Monitor BUN, serum creatinine, LDH, and bilirubin levels
Febrile, nonhemolytic Usually occurs within 30 min after initiation of transfusion to 6 hr after transfusion completed.	• Fever >1° C above baseline temperature • Flushing • Chills • Headache	• Stop transfusion • Administer antipyretics as ordered • Monitor temperature q4h
Allergic reaction—anaphylaxis Usually occurs within 5-15 min after initiation of transfusion.	• Hypotension • Decreased responsiveness • Severe dyspnea • Generalized edema may be present	• Stop transfusion • Airway and breathing support (anticipate intubation) • Administer epinephrine • Start NS or LR
Allergic reaction—mild to moderate Usually occurs during transfusion and up to 1 hr after transfusion completed.	• Urticaria • Pruritus • Hives • Facial edema • Fever • Nausea/vomiting • Dyspnea	• Stop transfusion • Administer antihistamine • Administer steroids • Administer acetaminophen

BUN, blood urea nitrogen; **LDH**, lactate dehydrogenase; **LR**, lactated Ringer's; **NS**, normal saline.

GASTROINTESTINAL

Insertion of a Nasogastric Tube[51]

Purpose: Gastric decompression or enteral feeding.

1. Place patient in a high-Fowler's position with pillows behind head and shoulders.

2. Assess nasal patency.

3. Determine length of tube to be inserted and mark with tape. For placement in stomach, measure distance from tip of nose, to earlobe, to xiphoid process of sternum.

4. Have patient tilt head back, lubricate tube and insert gently through nostril to back of throat (posterior nasopharynx). When tube reaches back of throat, allow patient to relax a moment and flex head towards chest.

5. Encourage patient to swallow tube. (If possible, give water with straw to facilitate swallowing.) Advance tube as patient swallows until desired length has been passed.

6. Check for position of tube in back of throat with tongue blade and penlight.

7. Check position of tube using Gastric pH.

   • With catheter-tip syringe, gently aspirate for gastric fluid; measure pH. Gastric pH ranges 1-4.

   • If tube is not in stomach, advance 2.5-5 cm (1-2 in) and again check position.

8. Secure tube to nose with tape or tube fixation device. Fasten tubing to patient gown.

9. Obtain x-ray to check final tube placement.

Administration of Enteral Nutrition (Tube Feeding)[52]

Purpose: Administration of nutrients via the GI tract for patients who are unable to eat, or who have increased energy requirements.

1. Assess type of tube used for enteral feeding (nasoenteric tube, gastrostomy tube, or jejunostomy tube).
2. Elevate patient's head of bed.
3. Verify tube placement, and measure residual.
   - Aspirate gastric secretions with syringe, noting volume and pH. Return aspirated contents and flush with 30 mL of water.
   - If aspirate volume >100 mL, do not return contents; hold feeding and notify physician (or per institutional policy).
   - If pH suggests improper placement of tube, hold feeding and notify physician.
4. Initiate feeding.
   - **Intermittent feeding:** Obtain desired amount of formula (room temperature).
     ▸ If using a feeding bag, place formula in bag and prime tubing. Attach distal end of tubing to proximal end of feeding tube; adjust rate of flow with roller clamp or a feeding pump. Infusion time varies depending on volume.
     ▸ If using a syringe, remove barrel of syringe and insert syringe tip into feeding tube. Pour desired amount of formula in upright syringe held 12-18 inches above insertion site. Allow formula to flow in by gravity.
     ▸ Upon completion of feeding, follow with 30-mL flush of water (or as specified), and clamp tubing.
     (continued)

- **Continuous feeding:**
  - ▶ Pour formula (no more than volume to be delivered in 4 hrs) in feeding bag and prime tubing. Connect tubing through feeding pump and attach distal end of tubing to proximal end of feeding tube. Set hourly rate and begin infusion. If new feeding, *gradually* work up to target infusion rate. Flush tube with 30 mL of water every 4-6 hrs.

5. Monitor for complications.
   - Intolerance of feeding (nausea, fullness, gastric residual >100 mL)
   - Aspiration of formula
   - Diarrhea more than 3 times in 24 hrs
   - Hyperglycemia (monitor glucose)
   - Fluid imbalance (monitor I&O)

GENITOURINARY

Insertion of a Urinary Catheter[51]

Purpose: Drainage of urine from the bladder.

1. Prepare patient.
   - Position patient (***female***—dorsal recumbent; ***male***—supine).
   - Drape to provide maximum modesty.
2. Set up equipment.
   - Open catheterization kit.
   - Don sterile gloves.
   - Organize supplies within kit.
3. Apply sterile drape, maintaining sterile technique.
   - ***Female:*** tuck under the buttocks.
   - ***Male:*** place over thighs just below the penis.

4. Clean urethral meatus.
   - *Female:* Spread labia with nondominant hand (maintain this position until catheter is inserted); pick up antiseptic swab with forceps; wipe from front to back (clitoris to anus) on each side of labia, then directly over center of urethral meatus (using a new swab for each wipe).
   - *Male:* Grasp penis at shaft just below glans with nondominant hand; pick up an antiseptic swab with forceps; clean tip of penis in circular motion from meatus down to base of glans—repeat at least 3 times (using a new swab each time).

5. Insert the catheter.
   - Pick up lubricated catheter with dominant hand and insert distal end through urethral meatus. Advance catheter until urine flows (*females* 2-3 in.; *males* 7-9 in.); upon flow, advance another 1-2 inches.
   - **Straight catheterization:** Drain urine from bladder using basin; when bladder is empty, remove catheter. (**Caution:** Follow agency policy regarding maximum amount of urine that can be drained at one time).
   - **Indwelling catheterization:** Inflate balloon and place drainage bag below level of bladder; secure catheter to patient's leg (*female*) or abdomen (*male*).

6. Complete procedure.
   - Remove supplies, document procedure noting color and volume of urine, and patient response to procedure.

Removal of an Indwelling Catheter[51]

1. Don clean gloves.
2. Withdraw all fluid from balloon with 10-mL syringe.
3. Gently pull catheter to remove; catch tip in a paper towel as it exits meatus to minimize urine leakage from the tip.
4. Empty urine bag. Dispose of catheter and urine bag in biohazard bag.

RESPIRATORY MANAGEMENT

Oxygen Delivery Devices[23]		
DEVICE	FLOW RATE (L/min)	% O_2 DELIVERED
Nasal cannula	1	24%
	2	28%
	3	32%
	4	36%
	5	40%
	6	44%
Simple mask	5-6	40%
	7-8	50%
	10	60%
Venturi mask*	Set per manufacture instructions- follow manufacture guidelines	24-50%
Partial rebreathing mask†	8-15	60-80%
Nonrebreathing mask†	8-15	80-100%
Oxymizer	1-6	28-46%
OxyMask	1-15	24-90%

*With use of appropriate entrainment port.
†Reservoir bag should never be fully collapsed.

Suctioning: Nasopharyngeal, Nasotracheal, Artificial Airway[51]

Purpose: Removal of mucus secretions from patient's airway and place pulse oximeter to monitor oxygenation during procedure.

1. Assess patient breath sounds.
2. Using aseptic technique, turn on suction device.
3. Open catheter package (size 10-16 French for adults) and fill basin with sterile saline solution.
4. Don sterile gloves and pick up sterile catheter with dominant hand; attach end to suction tubing.
5. Check equipment by suctioning small amount of saline from basin.
6. Hyperinflate and Hyperoxygenate the patient.
7. Insert catheter (without applying suction)
   Nasopharyngeal - insert catheter into nose about 6 inches in adults,
   Nasotracheal - insert catheter in nose about 8 inches in adults
   Artificial airway - insert catheter into artificial airway on inspiration until resistance is met or patient coughs.
8. Apply suction intermittently while slowly withdrawing the catheter in a rotating fashion.
9. Encourage patient to cough. Observe for respiratory distress.
10. Allow patient to recover and encourage deep breaths.
11. Clear catheter and tubing with normal saline.
12. Reassess patient after 1 minute; repeat suctioning up to two additional times as needed.

Assessment of a Patient with a Chest Tube[52]

Purpose: Removal of air or fluid from the pleural space.

- Assess patient's respiratory status
  Note the following:
  - ► Air movement bilaterally
  - ► Depth and effort of respirations
  - ► Oxygen saturation
  - ► Pain at chest tube insertion site
- Assess chest tube insertion site
  - ► Usually located in 5th or 6th intercostal space
  - ► Occlusive dressing over insertion site should be dry and intact
- Assess the chest tube drainage system
  - ► Type of system (water-seal or waterless system)
  - ► Volume, color, and consistency of drainage; measure drainage output once every shift or as indicated
  - ► Tidaling in water seal chamber (water seal system) or in diagnostic air leak indicator (waterless system); tidaling usually stops after 2-3 days once lung is reexpanded
  - ► Suction is at desired level
  - ► Look for possible air leak in system. Possible sources of air leak: patient or chest tube drainage system. Assess system by looking for constant bubbling in water seal chamber (water seal system) or constant bubbling in diagnostic air leak indicator (waterless system).

Pulse Oximetry: Interpretation and Action

FINDING	INTERPRETATION	ACTION
SaO_2 >94%	PaO_2 is >70 mm Hg	None; continue to monitor patient.
SaO_2 between 90%-94%	PaO_2 is between 60-70 mm Hg	No immediate action; may reposition probe; continue to monitor patient.
SaO_2 between 85%-90%	PaO_2 is between 50-60 mm Hg	Place patient in high-Fowler's or semi-Fowler's position; instruct patient to take slow deep breaths; prepare to administer oxygen (if not already in use); consider notifying physician depending on patient response.*
SaO_2 <85%	PaO_2 <50 mm Hg	Immediately administer oxygen; stay with patient; notify provider.

*Action may depend on patient's baseline saturation.

Performing a Dressing Change[54]

Purpose: Wound assessment; wound debridement.

1. Don clean gloves and remove tape, bandage, or ties.
2. Carefully remove dressings, taking care not to dislodge drains or tubes if present. Dispose of soiled dressings and gloves in a biohazard bag.
3. Assess wound appearance and color, odor, consistency, and amount (COCA) of drainage. Assess wound edges for degree of healing.
4. Obtain dressing supplies.
   - Open dressings.
   - For a wet-to-damp dressing, pour prescribed solution into sterile basin; add gauze.
5. Clean wound with prescribed antiseptic solution or normal saline if indicated. Clean from least contaminated to most contaminated area.
6. Apply dressing directly onto wound surface.
   - If wound is deep, pack gauze into wound with forceps until all wound surfaces are in contact with gauze.
7. Cover dressing with appropriate bandage (such as an ABD pad, Surgipad, or gauze) and secure as appropriate (tape, Montgomery straps, gauze roll, or other device).
8. Write date, time and initials on tape and apply to dressing.

VITAL SIGNS/ASSESSMENT

Clinical Findings of Common Conditions

SEE ALSO

OBSTETRICS

PEDIATRICS

Vital Signs—Adults[65]

VITAL SIGN AND RANGE*	METHOD OF MEASUREMENT
Temperature Oral 36.4°-37.6° C (97.6°-99.6° F) Tympanic 37.0°-38.1°C (98.6°-100.6° F) Rectal 37.0°-38.1°C (98.6°-100.6° F) Temporal Artery 37.0°-38.0° C (98.6°-100.4° F)	Measure with a thermometer: tympanic, electronic, temporal, or chemical (disposable). See temperature measurement chart on page 24.
Heart Rate 60-100 bpm	Palpate pulse, count number of pulsations per minute, or count number of auscultated heart sounds per minute.
Respiratory Rate 12-20 resp/min	Watching rise and fall of chest, count number of respirations per minute.
Oxygen Saturation ≥95%	Measure with pulse or ear pulse oximeter. Clip the probe (sensor) on the fingertip or earlobe.
Systolic 110-139 (Under 60 yrs of age) 110-149 (60 yrs or older) Diastolic 60-79 (under 60 yrs of age) 60-89 (60 yrs or older)	Measure with sphygmomanometer. BP determined through auscultation of Korotkoff sounds as cuff is deflated (noting when sounds begin and end).

*See normal pediatric ranges on p. 138.

Temperature Measurement Sites[52]

SITE	ADVANTAGES	DISADVANTAGES
Rectum	• Argued to be more reliable when one cannot obtain an oral temperature	• Measurement lag during rapid temp changes • Not used for patients with diarrhea/rectal problems, ↓ platelets • May be uncomfortable/embarrassing • Risk of exposure to body fluids
Oral	• Easy access • Provides accurate surface temperature reading • Reflects rapid change in core temperature • Reliable for intubated patients	• Affected by recent ingestion of hot/cold fluids or foods, smoking, oxygen therapy • Not used for patients with oral surgery/trauma/chills/epilepsy • Not used with infants/small children or confused/uncooperative patients • Risk of exposure to body fluids
Temporal artery	• Easy, safe access • Rapid measurement • Can be used with all ages • Reflects rapid change in core temperature	• Inaccurate with head covering or hair on forehead • Affected by skin moisture such as sweating
Tympanic membrane	• Easy, safe access • Rapid measurement • Accurate core reading	• Hearing aids must be removed • Requires disposable sensor cover and only one size available • Excess ear wax or infection can distort reading • Inaccurate reading with improper positioning of handheld unit • Not used for patients with ear surgery or injury or with children <3 yrs old

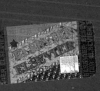

4e

MOSBY'S PDQ *for* RN

Nursing Facts at Hand

practical
Waterproof &
stain resistant

detailed
Key clinical facts,
including lab values,
assessment tools,
common drugs,
and much more

quick
Pocket-size
for instant access

ELSEVIER

Reviewers

Make this book work for you!

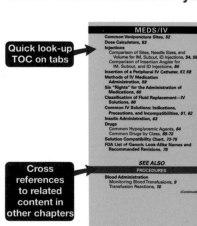

Quick look-up TOC on tabs →

Cross references to related content in other chapters →

MEDS/IV

(Continued)

Guidelines for Goal Blood Pressure in Adults with Hypertension[34]

PATIENT SUBGROUP	TARGET SBP (mm/Hg)	TARGET DBP (mm/Hg)
≥60 years of age	<150	<90
<60 years of age	<140	<90
>18 with CKD	<140	<90
>18 with diabetes	<140	<90

CKD, Chronic Kidney Disease.

Common Mistakes in Blood Pressure Measurement

ERROR	EFFECT
Bladder or cuff too wide	False low reading
Bladder or cuff too narrow	False high reading
Cuff wrapped too loosely	False high reading
Deflating cuff too slowly	False high diastolic
Deflating cuff too quickly	False low systolic and false high diastolic
Poorly fitting stethoscope ear pieces/Examiner hearing impairment	False low systolic and false high diastolic
Inaccurate inflation level	False low systolic
Arm unsupported	False high reading
Arm above heart	False low reading
Feet crossed when seated	False high reading

Basic Principles for Taking a Health History

- Introduce yourself; explain what is expected and time involved.
- Provide privacy.
- Communicate at appropriate level.
- Ask questions in a straightforward, non-judgmental manner.
- Use open-ended questions when possible.
- Actively listen to the patient.
- Maintain cultural sensitivity.
- Project warm, caring demeanor.
- Maintain professional interaction.

Components of a Symptom Analysis

Location: Where are the symptoms?

Quality: Describe symptom characteristics.

Quantity: Describe symptom severity.

Chronology: When did symptom start? How long does symptom last?

Setting: Where are you and what are you doing when symptom occurs?

Associated Manifestations: Presence of other symptoms?

Alleviating Factors: What makes symptom better?

Aggravating Factors: What makes symptom worse?

Components of a Health History

- Biographical data
- Chief complaint or presenting problem
- Medications/allergies
- Past health history
- Family history
- Social history
- Review of systems
  - **Integument:** rashes, sores, lesions, excessive dryness, bruising
  - **Head:** headaches, vertigo, syncope
  - **Eyes:** change in vision, pain, discharge, sensitivity to light
  - **Ears:** pain, discharge, change in hearing, tinnitus
  - **Nose and Sinuses:** epistaxis, obstruction, pain, discharge, snoring
  - **Mouth:** sore throat, bleeding gums, dysphagia, altered taste, lesions
  - **Neck:** enlarged lymph nodes, pain, stiffness
  - **Cardiovascular:** palpitations, chest pain, cold extremities, edema, paresthesia
  - **Respiratory:** cough, dyspnea, hemoptysis, pain, wheezing
  - **Gastrointestinal:** eating patterns, problems with digestion, abdominal pain, change in stools
  - **Urinary:** changes in urinary pattern, nocturia, dysuria, urgency, hesitancy
  - **Reproductive:** lesions, discharges, odors, pain, impotence (men), menstrual history (women)
  - **Musculoskeletal:** limitation or pain with movement, gait, joint swelling, muscle weakness
  - **Neurologic:** cognitive changes, seizures, paralysis, paresthesia

Pain Assessment[65]

Onset	When does pain occur? During activity? Before/after eating? Sudden/ gradual?
Location	Where is the pain located?
Duration	How long does it last? Is it constant or intermittent?
Characteristics	What does the pain feel like? (eg: dull, sharp, throbbing)
Aggravating Factors	What makes the pain worse? (eg: moving, standing, sitting)?
Related Symptoms	What other signs/symptoms accompany the pain (eg: SOB, rapid breathing, palpitations, sweating, nausea, vomiting)
Treatment by Patient	How have you tried to relieve the pain? How effective have these measures been?
Severity	How severe is your pain? (see pain rating scale)
Observed Behaviors	What behaviors are displayed? (eg: agitation, crying, moaning, restlessness, rubbing, guarding)

Numeric Pain Intensity Scale

0----1----2----3----4----5----6----7----8----9----10

No Pain	Moderate Pain	Worst Pain

Substance-Abuse Screening: CAGE

The four-item CAGE questionnaire is one of the simplest and most commonly used screening tools for substance use disorders.

CAGE Questions

C "Have you ever felt you ought to **Cut** down on your drinking or drug use?"

A "Have people **Annoyed** you by criticizing your drinking or drug use?"

G "Have you felt bad or **Guilty** about your drinking or drug use?"

E "Have you ever had a drink or used drugs first thing in the morning to steady your nerves or to get rid of a hangover (**Eye-opener**)?"

US Standard Drink Equivalents[48]

12 oz. of beer or cooler	8-9 oz. of malt liquor 8.5 oz. shown in a 12-oz. glass that, if full, would hold about 1.5 standard drinks of malt liquor	5 oz. of table wine	1.5 oz. of spirits (a single jigger of 80-proof gin, vodka, whiskey, etc.) Shown straight and in a highball glass with ice to show level before adding mixer*
12 oz.	8.5 oz.	5 oz.	1.5 oz.

Woman Abuse Screening Tool (WAST)[15]

1. In general, how would you describe your relationship?	3- lot of tension 2- some tension 1- no tension
2. Do you and your partner work out arguments with:	3- great difficulty 2- some difficulty 1- no difficulty
3. Do arguments ever result in you feeling down or bad about yourself?	3- often 2- sometimes 1- never
4. Do arguments ever result in hitting, kicking, or pushing?	3- often 2- sometimes 1- never
5. Do you ever feel frightened by what your partner says or does?	3- often 2- sometimes 1- never
6. Has your partner ever abused you physically?	3- often 2- sometimes 1- never
7. Has your partner ever abused you emotionally?	3- often 2- sometimes 1- never
8. Has your partner ever abused you sexually?	3- often 2- sometimes 1- never

Score of 13 or higher is considered an indicator of IPV.

Components of a Basic Examination[65]

AREA	EXAMINATION
General survey	Note overall appearance, including skin color, posture, facial expression, nutrition status, hygiene, gait, etc.
Mental status	Assess level of consciousness; orientation to person, place, and time; and emotional affect.
Head/neck	Assess shape of head, characteristics of hair and skin, presence of lesions, facial symmetry, eye movement, pupils, visual acuity, hearing, nasal patency and drainage, condition of teeth and mucous membranes, lesions, ROM of neck, lymph nodes, thyroid enlargement, carotid pulses.
Chest	Inspect respiratory effort, chest shape and movement, skin characteristics, breasts, spine. Auscultate breath sounds (anterior, lateral, posterior) and heart sounds.
Abdomen	Inspect contour, movement, skin characteristics and lesions. Auscultate for bowel sounds in four quadrants. Light palpation to determine firmness, distention, and presence of pain; deep palpation for masses.
Extremities	Assess ROM in all extremities; symmetry, muscle strength, presence of deformities; quality of pulses, capillary refill, skin characteristics, presence of lesions, hair distribution, presence of edema, temperature, color.
Genitalia/perineum	Inspect hygiene, skin condition, presence of lesions, drainage, etc.

Respiratory System

Assessments

Depth: Deep or shallow
Rhythm: Even or uneven
Effort: Ease, quiet, or with great effort
Expansion: Symmetric or asymmetric
Cough: Productive, nonproductive, or absent
Auscultation: Air exchange throughout lungs; presence of adventitious sounds (crackles, wheezes, rubs); presence of diminished, lowered, or distant sounds; absence of sounds

Auscultation and Percussion Sites[55]

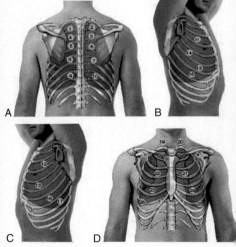

Suggested sequence for systematic percussion and auscultation of the thorax. **A,** Posterior thorax. **B,** Right lateral thorax. **C,** Left lateral thorax. **D,** Anterior thorax. The pleximeter finger or the stethoscope is moved in the numeric sequence suggested.

Patterns of Respiration

Normal

Regular and comfortable at a rate of 12-20 breaths per minute

Bradypnea

Slower than 12 breaths per minute

Tachypnea

Faster than 20 breaths per minute

Hyperventilation (hyperpnea)

Faster than 20 breaths per minute, deep breathing

Sighing

Frequently interspersed deeper breath

Air trapping

Increasing difficulty in getting breath out

Cheyne-Stokes

Varying periods of increasing depth interspersed with apnea

Kussmaul

Rapid, deep, labored

Biot

Irregularly interspersed periods of apnea in a disorganized sequence of breaths

Ataxic

Significant disorganization with irregular and varying depths of respiration

Cardiovascular System

Areas of Heart Auscultation[55]

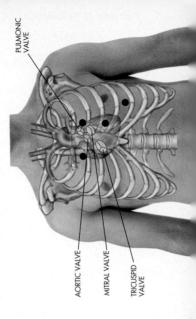

PULMONIC VALVE

AORTIC VALVE

MITRAL VALVE

TRICUSPID VALVE

- The aortic area—second right intercostal space (ICS) right sternal border (RSB)
- The pulmonic area—second left ICS left sternal border (LSB)
- The tricuspid area—fourth left ICS LSB
- The mitral area—fifth left ICS midclavicular line

Note: Black circles indicate placement of stethoscope.

Assessment of Peripheral Perfusion

Pulse Scale:
0   Absent
1+ Diminished, barely palpable, easy to obliterate
2+ Easily palpable
3+ Full pulse, increased
4+ Strong, bounding, cannot be obliterated

Color: Skin tone, pinkish, cyanotic, red, pallor

Swelling/edema: See pitting edema scale on
next page.

Skin: Appearance of skin, presence of hair,
presence of lesions

Pain/paresthesia: Presence of pain; sensation
and movement

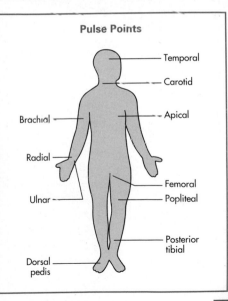

Pulse Points

Temporal
Carotid
Brachial
Apical
Radial
Ulnar
Femoral
Popliteal
Posterior tibial
Dorsal pedis

Assessment Scale for Pitting Edema

1+ Slight pitting, no visible distortion, disappears rapidly

2 mm

2+ Somewhat deeper pit than in 1+, no readily detectable distortion, disappears in 10-15 sec

4 mm

3+ Pit noticeably deep, may last more than a minute; the dependent extremity looks fuller and swollen

6 mm

4+ Pit very deep, lasts 2-5 min; dependent extremity is grossly distorted

8 mm

Integument System

Components of Skin Assessment

- Color (pink, reddish, tan, brown, pale, cyanotic, jaundice)
- Temperature (cold, cool, warm, hot)
- Moisture (dry, moist, diaphoretic)
- Turgor (rapid, slow)
- Lesion(s) (describe location, size, color, shape, borders, elevation, grouping)
- Edema

Pressure Points for Pressure Ulcer Development[61]

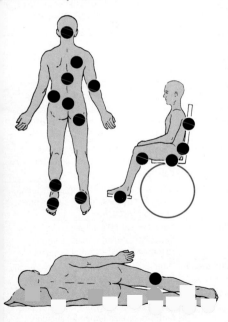

Musculoskeletal System

Muscle Strength Scale	
0	No detection of muscular contraction
1	A barely detectable flicker or trace of contraction with observation or palpation
2	Active movement of body part with elimination of gravity
3	Active movement against gravity only and not against resistance
4	Active movement against gravity and some resistance
5	Active movement against full resistance without evident fatigue (normal muscle strength)

Neurologic System

Level of Consciousness Assessment Terms	
Alert	Awake, oriented, converses and responds appropriately.
Confused	Disorientation, restless, agitated, difficulty following commands, memory deficits.
Lethargy	Oriented, but slowed mental responses. Speech may be sluggish, sleeps often, but easily arousable.
Obtunded	Very drowsy, falls asleep easily, more difficult to awaken. Limited verbal responses, follows simple commands.
Stuporous	Difficult to arouse, only awakens briefly. Displays very little motor movement.
Coma	Does not arouse, does not respond to verbal stimuli. May or may not display motor response to painful stimulus.

Glasgow Coma Scale		
ACTION	**BEST RESPONSE**	**SCORE**
Eyes open	Spontaneously	4
	To speech	3
	To pain	2
	None	1
Verbal	Oriented	5
	Confused	4
	Inappropriate words	3
	Incomprehensible sounds	2
	None	1
Motor	Obeys commands	6
	Localized pain	5
	Flexion withdrawal	4
	Abnormal flexion	3
	Abnormal extension	2
	Flaccid	1
Total		**15**

Pupillary Size in Millimeters

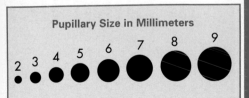

Cranial Nerve Functions

CRANIAL NERVE		SENSORY OR MOTOR FUNCTION
I	Olfactory	**Sensory:** Smell reception and interpretation
II	Optic	**Sensory:** Visual acuity and visual fields
III	Oculomotor	**Motor:** Extraocular eye movements, elevation of lids, pupillary constriction, control of lens shape
IV	Trochlear	**Motor:** Downward and inward eye movement
V	Trigeminal	**Sensory:** Sensation of face, scalp, cornea, oral and nasal mucous membranes **Motor:** Chewing movements of the jaw
VI	Abducens	**Motor:** Lateral eye movement
VII	Facial	**Sensory:** Taste on the anterior 2/3 of the tongue **Motor:** Facial movement, eye closure, labial speech
VIII	Acoustic	**Sensory:** Hearing and balance
IX	Glossopharyngeal	**Sensory:** Taste on the posterior 1/3 of the tongue, pharyngeal gag reflex, sensation from the eardrum and ear canal **Motor:** Swallowing and phonation muscles of the pharynx
X	Vagus	**Sensory:** Sensation from pharynx, viscera, carotid body, and carotid sinus **Motor:** Swallowing and talking muscles of the palate, pharynx, and larynx
XI	Spinal Accessory	**Motor:** Trapezius and sternocleidomastoid muscle movement
XII	Hypoglossal	**Motor:** Tongue movement for speech, sound articulation, and swallowing

CLINICAL FINDINGS OF COMMON CONDITIONS

Common Communicable Diseases of the Skin

DISEASE	INCUBATION	INTEGUMENT FINDINGS
Herpes simplex virus	2-12 days	Lesions appear on upper lip or on genitalia. Initial symptoms are stinging and increased sensitivity followed by lesions that progress from vesicles, to pustule, to crust.
Impetigo	N/A	Highly contagious; bacterial infection; vesicular lesions; advances to yellow crust on a red base.
Lice (pediculosis)	Eggs hatch in 7 days	Infestation of body hair; transmitted by direct contact with infested person; eggs and nits can be seen in hair attached to hair shaft.
Scabies	2-6 weeks	Infestation of skin; transmission by direct contact; mite penetration is visible as papules or vesicles or as tiny, linear burrows containing mites and their eggs; causes intense itching.
Lyme disease	3-32 days after tick exposure	Tick-borne spirochetal disease; distinctive circular red skin lesion with central clearing; accompanied by malaise, fatigue, fever, headache, stiff neck, arthralgias, or lymphadenopathy.

Characteristics of Headaches

TYPE	DESCRIPTION
Migraine headache	Headache starts with aura. Unilateral pain lasts 2-72 hrs. Associated symptoms: photophobia, irritability, nausea, vomiting, and depression. Occurs 2 times more frequently in women; frequency decreases with advanced age.
Cluster headache	Closely grouped headache attacks over period of days or weeks. Described as burning or stabbing unilateral pain behind eye lasting 1/2 to 1 hr. Associated symptoms: facial flushing, nasal congestion, ptosis, lacrimation, rhinorrhea, and salivation. Occurs 4 times more often in men; generally occurs in 3rd and 4th decades of life.
Tension headache	Bilateral headache usually diffuse or confined to frontal, temporal, parietal, or occipital area; often described as tight band around head. Onset is usually gradual and lasts several days. Most common type of headache in persons ages 20-40.

Lung Conditions and Expected Sounds[39]

TYPE	DESCRIPTION
Pneumonia and consolidation	Bronchovesicular or bronchial breath sounds over the affected area. Crackles may be present on late inspiration.
Pneumothorax	Decreased or absent breath sounds. No adventitious sounds present.
Tumor	Decreased or absent breath sounds over area.
Emphysema	Bronchial breath sounds with prolonged expiration and decreased intensity. Fine crackles often present in late inspiration; occasional rhonchi heard.
Pleural effusion	Decreased or absent breath sounds. A pleural friction rub may be heard.
Asthma	Bronchovesicular breath sounds. Wheezes or sibilant rhonchi usually present.
Atelectasis	Vesicular breath sounds. Crackles may be heard in late inspiration.
Bronchitis	Vesicular breath sounds. Crackles and sibilant rhonchi present.

Clinical Manifestations of Electrolyte Imbalance[25]

IMBALANCE	CLINICAL MANIFESTATIONS	CAUSES
Hyponatremia Na <135 mEq/L	Fatigue, abdominal cramps, diarrhea, weakness, hypotension, cool clammy skin	Excess sweating, excess intake of water, diuretics, adrenal insufficiency, renal failure
Hypernatremia Na >145 mEq/L	Thirst; dry, sticky mucous membranes; dry tongue and skin; flushed skin; increased temperature	Diarrhea, decreased water intake, saltwater ingestion, impaired renal function, febrile illness, inability to swallow, burns, diabetes insipidus
Hypokalemia K <3.5 mEq/L	Weakness, fatigue, anorexia, abdominal distention, cardiac arrhythmias	Diarrhea, vomiting, diuretics, burns, heat stress, ulcerative colitis, potassium-free IV fluids, metabolic acidosis, steroids
Hyperkalemia K >5.0 mEq/L	Cardiac arrhythmias, anxiety, increased bowel sounds, abdominal cramps	Acute/chronic renal failure, burns, crush injuries, metabolic acidosis, potassium-sparing diuretics
Hypocalcemia Ca <4.5 mg/dL	Abdominal cramps, tingling, muscle spasm, convulsions	Parathyroid dysfunction, vitamin D deficiency, pancreatitis
Hypercalcemia Ca >5.6 mg/dL	Bone pain, nausea, vomiting, constipation	Parathyroid tumor, bone cancer/metastasis, osteoporosis

Acid-Base Imbalances[50]

RESPIRATORY ACIDOSIS

Causes: Carbonic acid excess usually resulting from respiratory compromise/failure

	Uncompensated	Compensated
pH	<7.35	Normal
PCO2	↑	↑

RESPIRATORY ALKALOSIS

Causes: Carbonic acid deficit usually resulting from hyperventilation

	Uncompensated	Compensated
pH	>7.35	Normal
PCO2	↓	↓

METABOLIC ACIDOSIS

Causes: Bicarbonate deficit due to renal failure, starvation, etc.

	Uncompensated	Compensated
pH	<7.35	Normal
PCO2	Normal	↓

METABOLIC ALKALOSIS

Causes: Bicarbonate excess due to hyperkalemia, excessive vomiting, diuretics, etc.

	Uncompensated	Compensated
pH	>7.35	Normal
PCO2	Normal	↑

Clinical Manifestations of Thyroid Gland Dysfunction[53]

Hyperthyroidism

- Increased body metabolism
- Nervousness/restlessness
- Short attention span
- Tachycardia (>100 bpm; bounding heart sounds)
- Increased blood pressure
- Reduced vital capacity
- Skin warm, moist, and smooth
- Hair fine, nails soft
- Weakness and fatigue
- Demineralization of bones
- Hypercalcemia
- Brisk reflexes
- Increased appetite/weight loss
- Muscle wasting
- Diabetes worsens
- Increased stools
- Increased libido
- Decreased fertility
- Higher body temperature

Hypothyroidism

- Decreased body metabolism
- Lethargy and headaches
- Memory deficit
- Bradycardia (<60 bpm; weak heart sounds)
- Decreased blood pressure
- Lowered respiratory rate
- Skin cool, dry, and rough
- Hair coarse, nails brittle
- Weakness and fatigue
- Stiff joints
- Mild proteinuria
- Decreased reflexes
- Decreased appetite/weight gain
- Muscular stiffness
- Diabetics need less insulin
- Constipation
- Decreased libido
- Decreased fertility
- Lower body temperature

Clinical Comparisons of Hypoglycemia and Hyperglycemia

	Hypoglycemia	Hyperglycemia
	<60 mg/dL	>250 mg/dL
Cause	• Too much insulin • Skipped or delayed meals • Too much exercise	• Too little insulin • Overeating • Emotional stress, illness, infection, surgery, stroke, heart attack, pregnancy • Ketoacidosis
Early symptoms	• Sweatiness, shakiness, weakness • Headache, dizziness • Hunger	• Excessive thirst • Frequent urination • Fatigue, weakness
Late symptoms	• Numbness of lips/tongue • Difficulty concentrating • Mood change/irritability • Vision changes, pallor • If not treated— seizures, coma	• Abdominal pain, nausea, vomiting • General aches, loss of appetite • Flushed, dry skin • Fruity breath, drowsiness • If not treated— labored breathing, coma

Signs and Symptoms of Prostate Enlargement or Cancer

- Weak or interrupted urine flow
- Difficulty starting or stopping urinary stream
- Inability to urinate
- Frequency, especially at night
- Hematuria
- Pain or burning on urination
- Constant pain in the lower back, pelvis, or upper thighs

Sexually Transmitted Infections[65]

INFECTION	CAUSE	SYMPTOMS
Chlamydia	*Chlamydia trachomatis*	♀ 75% asymptomatic; painful frequent urination, vaginal bleeding/ discharge ♂ urethral discharge, dysuria, itching
Gonorrhea	*Neisseria gonorrhoeae*	♀ yellow/green vaginal discharge, dysuria, pelvic pain, irregular menses ♂ penile discharge, urethritis, dysuria
Syphilis	*Treponema pallidum*	Primary lesion—single painless ulcer on genitalia or mouth; Secondary lesion—skin rash; flat, oval, or round grayish lesions
Trichomoniasis	*Trichomonas vaginalis*	♀ malodorous greenish yellow vaginal discharge, vulvar irritation
Herpes Genitalis	HSV2	Burning on urination, genital pain, fever, genital vesicles that ulcerate on rupture More common & severe in women
Genital warts	HPV*	Soft pink to brown lesions on internal & external genital & anal areas
Lice/crabs	*Pediculosis pubis*	Intense itching, nits/lice seen in pubic hair
HIV**	HIV-1&2	Asymptomatic for years; symptoms develop after immune system weakens

HSV2, herpes simplex virus; **HPV,** human papillomavirus; **HIV,** human immunodeficiency virus;
*Note: CDC recommends HPV vaccine for all female and male preteens to prevent warts & possible cancer.
**Note: HIV Screening recommended for all persons seeking treatment for STDs.
See www.cdc.gov/hpv/vaccine.html for additional information.

MEDS/IV

SEE ALSO

PROCEDURES

EMERGENCY/ECG

(Continued)

Meds/IV

Meds/IV

MEDS/IV

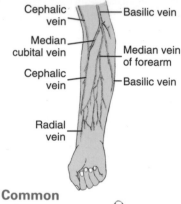

Common Venipuncture Sites[52]

Cephalic vein — Basilic vein

Median cubital vein — Median vein of forearm

Cephalic vein — Basilic vein

Radial vein

Superficial dorsal veins

Dorsal venous arch

Cephalic vein — Basilic vein

DOSE CALCULATORS

Dosages

$$\frac{\text{Dose ordered}}{\text{Dose on hand}} = \text{Amount to administer}$$

Example: Tablet $\dfrac{15 \text{ mg}}{5 \text{ mg/tablet}} = 3$ tablets

Liquid $\dfrac{35 \text{ mg}}{50 \text{ mg/mL}} = 0.7$ mL

Solution Concentration

$$\frac{\text{Dosage in solution}}{\text{Volume of solution}} = \text{Solution concentration}$$

Example: $\dfrac{100 \text{ mg}}{500 \text{ mL}} = 0.2$ mg/ml

IV Dose Rate Calculation

$$\frac{\text{Dose ordered}}{\text{Solution concentration}} = \text{Volume/hour}$$

Example: $\dfrac{50 \text{ mg/hr}}{2 \text{ mg/mL}} = 25$ mL/hr

Comparison of Sites, Needle Sizes, and Volume for IM, Sub-Q, ID Injections[22]

TYPE: IM **NEEDLE SIZE** 23-25 G 5/8"-1" **VOLUME** **Average** 0.5 ml **Range** 0.5-2 ml	**SITE:** Deltoid muscle[29] 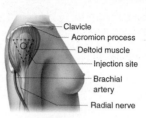 - Clavicle - Acromion process - Deltoid muscle - Injection site - Brachial artery - Radial nerve
TYPE: IM **NEEDLE SIZE** 20-23 G 1½"-3" **VOLUME** **Average** 2 ml **Range** 1-5 ml	**SITE:** Ventrogluteal muscle[29] 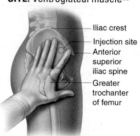 - Iliac crest - Injection site - Anterior superior iliac spine - Greater trochanter of femur
TYPE: IM **NEEDLE SIZE** 20-23 G 1½"-3" **VOLUME** **Average** 2 ml **Range** 1-5 ml	**SITE:** Dorsogluteal muscle[29] 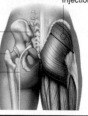 - Injection site - Posterior superior iliac spine - Greater trochanter of femur - Sciatic nerve

TYPE: IM
NEEDLE SIZE
22-25 G
$5/8''$–$1 1/2''$

VOLUME
Average
2 ml
Range
1-5 ml

SITE: Vastus lateralis muscle[29]

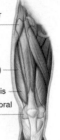

Greater
trochanter
of femur

Injection site
(middle third)

Vastus lateralis

Lateral femoral
condyle

TYPE: SC
NEEDLE SIZE
25-27 G
$1/2''$-$5/8''$

VOLUME
Average
0.5 ml
Range
0.5-1.5 ml

SITE: Arm, abdomen, thigh[29]

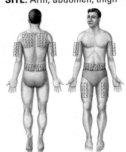

TYPE: ID
NEEDLE SIZE
26-27 G
$3/8''$

VOLUME
Average
0.1 ml
Range
0.001-1.0 ml

SITE: Forearm[29]

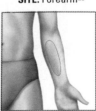

Comparison of Insertion Angles for IM, SC, and ID Injections[52]

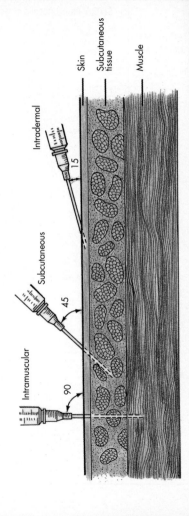

Intramuscular   Subcutaneous   Intradermal

90   45   15

Skin

Subcutaneous
tissue

Muscle

54

Z-Track Injection[29]

Purpose: Prevents seepage of medication through injection track with an IM injection.

1. Prepare injection.
2. Select site.
3. Clean skin with alcohol.
4. Slide skin to side 1.0–1.5 in.
5. Inject medication at 90-degree angle.
6. Withdraw needle.
7. Release skin.

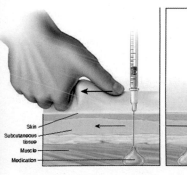
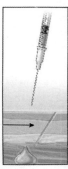

Skin
Subcutaneous tissue
Muscle
Medication

Insertion of a Peripheral Intravenous Catheter[52]
(Over-the-Needle Catheter)

Purpose: Peripheral IV access for administration of fluids and/or medications.

1. Select venipuncture site.

2. Clean site using circular motion with 2% chlorhexidine.

3. Apply tourniquet.

4. Anchor vein by stretching skin; insert needle bevel up at 20- to 30-degree angle.

5. Watch for blood return in flashback chamber of the catheter.

6. Advance needle another ¼ inch; then advance catheter into the vein until hub is at the venipuncture site.

7. Stabilize catheter and release tourniquet.

8. Remove needle stylet and attach tubing or saline lock to catheter hub. Flush with saline to verify patency.

9. Secure catheter and apply sterile dressing (gauze or transparent) to site.

Advance Device into Vein[52]

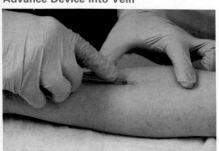

Types of Care for a Central Line Catheter

Purpose: Delivery of all types of IV medications, fluids, blood products; drawing blood. Tip of catheter lies in the central venous system.

1. Types of central line catheters:
   - **Peripherally Inserted Central Catheter (PICC):** Percutaneously inserted through skin into vein in antecubital fossa and threaded until tip in central venous system. Usually long-term placement.
   - **Central Venous Catheter:** At bedside; usually inserted directly through skin into large vein in neck; threaded into superior vena cava. Usually short-term placement.
   - **Hickman, Broviac, Groshong Catheters:** Surgically inserted in cephalic or jugular veins; threaded into superior vena cava. Catheter tunneled under skin, exits on upper chest. Usually long-term placement.
   - **Implanted Port:** Surgically inserted in cephalic or jugular veins and threaded into superior vena cava. Catheter attached to port with diaphragm. Port planted in chest tissue; skin acts as protective covering. Usually long-term placement.

2. Care guidelines
   - **Dressings:** Sterile gauze or transparent occlusion dressing.
   - **Flush:** Lines must be flushed with NaCl before and NaCl and heparin after each use, or every 12-24 hrs when not in use. (Groshong lines do not use heparin.)
   - **Access:** Most central line catheters are accessed through an injection cap. Implanted port accessed by inserting noncoring needle through skin into port.
   - **Assessment:** Monitor patient for fever, redness/swelling/discharge at site. If catheter has a clamp, be sure it is on if line is not in use.

Methods of IV Medication Administration

METHOD AND DESCRIPTION	ACCESS
IV Push Medication drawn up in syringe (undiluted or diluted) and administered over an appropriate time (usually less than 5 minutes).	**Saline Lock:** Clean port, flush with 1-2 mL NaCl; administer medication over desired time; follow with 1-2 mL NaCl flush. **Primary Line:** Clean most distal injection port on primary line (closest to patient); administer medication into IV line over desired time.
Intermittent IV Medication Infusion Medication added to small (e.g., 50-100 mL) IV bag and infused over specified time frame (e.g., 30 min to 1 hr) at designated intervals. If given through a primary line, referred to as "IV piggyback (IVPB)."	**Saline Lock:** Clean port, flush with 1-2 mL NaCl; attach IV tubing to port; open roller clamp and infuse at desired rate. After infusion, remove tubing and flush port with 1-2 mL of NaCl. **Primary Line:** Hang IVPB higher than primary IV; clean proximal injection port on primary line; insert IVPB; open roller clamp; infuse at desired rate. After IVPB is completed, and primary IV begins to infuse, remove IVPB set.
Continuous IV Medication Infusion Medication is mixed in specified type and volume of IV fluid (usually 250 mL or more) and administered continuously at specified dosage rate.	**As a Primary Line:** Set rate of infusion as specified. Continuous IV medication infusions are typically regulated on IV pump. **Through a Primary Line:** Continuous IV medication infusion may be delivered through another primary IV line. Both infusions run at same time at independent infusion rates.

Six "Rights" for the Administration of Medication

Right drug	Determine accuracy of order. If order seems incorrect, consult prescriber before administering.
Right dose	Double check drug calculations. When unsure of calculations, get a second opinion.
Right patient	Verify patient's identity by checking ID band and asking patient to state name.
Right route	Administer drugs by their prescribed route.
Right time	Follow agency's routine medication administration schedule. Stat orders should be given immediately.
Right documentation	Promptly chart medication administration on the right record for the right time.

Nurse's Six Rights for Safe Medication Administration[44]

1. The right to a complete and clearly written order that clearly specifies the drug, dose, route, and frequency.
2. The right to have the correct drug route and dose dispensed.
3. The right to have access to drug information.
4. The right to have policies on safe medication Administration.
5. The right to administer medications safely and to identify problems in the system
6. The right to stop, think, and be vigilant when administering medications.

Common IV Solutions: Indications, Precautions, and Incompatibilities[21]

SOLUTION/TYPE	INDICATIONS	PRECAUTIONS	INCOMPATIBILITIES
D5W Hypotonic	Replace water and low calorie needs Dehydration Hyperkalemia Spares body protein; provides nutrition	Do not use in head trauma, in early postoperative patients, or in patients with fluid overload (CHF) Contraindicated with diabetes	Whole blood Ampicillin Erythromycin Warfarin Fat emulsions Sodium bicarbonate Dilantin B_{12}
0.9% saline Isotonic	Replace ECF Hyponatremia Hypochloremia Water overload Mild metabolic acidosis Medication diluent IV irrigant Compatible with blood	Does not contain any free water or calories Can cause fluid overload, hypokalemia, hypernatremia, hyperchloremic acidosis Use caution with renal or circulatory impairment, older adults, and those with sodium retention	Amphotericin B Mannitol Diazepam Fat emulsions Chlordiazepoxide Methylprednisolone Warfarin Whole blood Ampicillin Erythromycin

D5/0.45 NS Hypertonic	Rehydrate; has free water, salt, and calories	Use caution with CHF, pulmonary edema, urinary obstruction, steroid therapy May falsely ↑ BUN Contraindicated in diabetic coma	Amphotericin B Mannitol Diazepam
Ringer's Isotonic	Replacement of fluid and electrolytes (dehydration, vomiting, diarrhea, burns) Volume expander Contains no calories	Do not use with CHF, renal insufficiency, or sodium retention Not enough potassium or calcium to be used as maintenance fluid	Ampicillin Cefamandole Diazepam Erythromycin Methicillin Potassium Phosphate Sodium bicarbonate Whole blood
Lactated Ringer's Isotonic	Resembles blood serum No free water Rehydration Burns, dehydration, DKA, salicylate overdose	Can cause hyperkalemia, hypernatremia Can exacerbate CHF, edema, and Na retention Contraindicated with liver disease, Addison's disease, severe metabolic acidosis and alkalosis, profound hypovolemia and hyperkalemia	Ampicillin Cefamandole Diazepam Erythromycin Phosphate Sodium bicarbonate

urea nitrogen; **CHF**, congestive heart failure; **DKA**, diabetic ketoacidosis; **ECF**, extracellular fluid; **IV**, intravenous; **Na**, sodium; **NS**, normal saline.

Insulin Administration[37]

Insulin Injection Tips
- Examine insulin before injection
  - Do not use past expiration date
  - Do not use if discolored/lumpy
- Select correct sub-q injection site
- Use short needle (4-5 mm)
- Inject at 90 degree angle
- Properly dispose of needle/syringe
- Rotate insulin sites weekly
- Store unopened insulin in refrigerator

Sites for Insulin Injection[37]

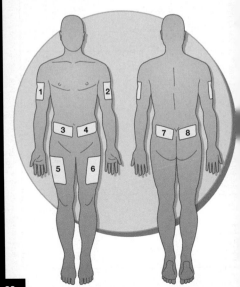

Common Hypoglycemic Agents[37]

TYPES	PEAK (hr)	DURATION (hr)
Oral agents		
Chlorpropamide (Diabinese)	1	24-60
Tolbutamide (Orinase)	5-8	6-12
Tolazamide (Tolinase)	4-6	12-24
Glipizide (Glucotrol)	1-3	10-24
Glyburide (DiaBeta, Micronase, Glynase PresTab)	2-8	24
Acarbose (Precose)	1	14-24
Acetohexamide (Dymelor)	1.3-8	12-24
Glimepiride (Amaryl)	2-3	24
Metformin hydrochloride (Glucophage)	1-3	9-17
Miglitol (Glyset)	2-3	24
Nateglinide (Starlix)	0-1	2-3
Repaglinide (Prandin)	1-1.5	<4
Insulin		
Rapid acting (onset 1 hr)		
Regular	2-4	4-12
Insulin zinc (Semilente)	5-10	12-16
Regular human (Humulin-R, Novolin-R)	1-3	3-5
Intermediate acting (onset 2-4 hr)		
Globin zinc (Iletin)	6-10	18-24
Isophane suspension (NPH)	4-12	18-24
Insulin zinc suspension (Iletin Lente)	7-15	18-24
NPH human isophane (Humulin-N, Novolin-N)	8-12	26-30
Long acting (onset 4-6 hr)		
Protamine zinc (PZ)	14-24	24-36
Insulin zinc extended (Ultralente)	10-30	>36
Insulin glargine (Lantus)	N/A	24

N/A, not applicable; **NPH**, neutral protein Hagedorn.

Common Prescription Drugs by Class[38]

COMMON DRUGS	TYPICAL ADULT DOSES	COMMON SIDE EFFECTS
Analgesics		
Celecoxib (Celebrex)	200 mg/bid	Diarrhea, heartburn, headache, URI
Naproxen (Aleve), Naprosyn	500-1250 mg/day	Nausea, constipation, cramps, heartburn, dizziness, drowsiness, headache
Tramadol (Ultram)	50-100 mg/q4-6h	Dizziness, vertigo, nausea, constipation, headache, drowsiness
Antianxiety		
Alprazolam (Xanax)	0.75-10 mg/day	Drowsiness, weakness, ataxia, slurred speech, confusion, nausea, lack of coordination, impaired memory, agitation, dizziness
Diazepam (Valium)	2-40 mg/day	Same for all antianxiety medications listed
Lorazepam (Ativan)	0.5-10 mg/day	Same for all antianxiety medications listed
Antibiotics		
Amoxicillin (Amoxil)	0.75-1.5 g/day	Diarrhea, nausea, vomiting, headaches, sore mouth/tongue, vaginal itching/discharge, allergic reaction (e.g., anaphylaxis, skin rash, hives, itching)
Amoxicillin/clavulanate (Augmentin)	250-500 mg/q 8 hr	Diarrhea, allergic reaction (e.g., anaphylaxis, skin rash, hives, itching)
Azithromycin (Zithromax)	PO: 500 mg on day 1, 250 mg on days 2-5	PO: Nausea, diarrhea, vomiting, abdominal pain IV: Pain, redness, swelling at injection site

Cephalexin (Keflex)	250-1000 mg/q6h	Sore mouth/tongue, diarrhea, abdominal cramps, vaginal itching/discharge
Doxycycline (Vibramycin)	100-200 mg/day	Anorexia, nausea, vomiting, diarrhea, dysphagia, photosensitivity
Ciprofloxacin (Cipro)	PO: 250-750 mg q12h IV: 200-400 mg q12h	Dizziness, headaches, nervousness, drowsiness, insomnia, abdominal pain, nausea, diarrhea, vomiting
Sulfamethoxazole-trimethoprim (Bactrim, Septra)	1 double strength tab/q 12-24h	Anorexia, nausea, vomiting, rash.itching
Anticoagulants/antiplatelets		
Clopidogrel (Plavix)	75 mg/day	Skin disorders
Heparin	DVT prophylaxis: 5000 units q8-12h DVT embolism: IV bolus, then IV infusion 20,000-40,000 units/day	Bleeding
Warfarin (Coumadin)	Initial: 5-10 mg, then 2-10 mg/day	Bleeding
Anticonvulsants		
Carbamazepine (Tegretol)	800-1200 mg/day	Vertigo, sleepiness, ataxia, fatigue, rash, itching, nausea, vomiting, leukopenia

continued

Common Drugs by Class (continued)

COMMON DRUGS	TYPICAL ADULT DOSES	COMMON SIDE EFFECTS
Clonazepam (Klonopin)	1.5-20 mg/day	Drowsiness, ataxia, agitation, irritability
Gabapentin (Neurontin)	300 mg/1-3 times a day	Fatigue, drowsiness, dizziness, ataxia
Pregabalin (Lyrica)	50 mg/3 times a day	Dizziness, drowsiness, ataxia, peripheral edema
Antidepressants		
Amitriptyline (Elavil)	40-300 mg/day	Drowsiness, blurred vision, constipation, confusion, postural hypotension, weight gain, seizure tendency
Citalopram (Celexa)	20 mg/day	Nausea, dry mouth, drowsiness, insomnia, sweating
Duloxetine (Cymbalta)	40-60 mg/day	Nausea, dry mouth, constipation, decreased appetite, fatigue, sweating
Escitalopram (Lexapro)	10 mg/day	Nausea, dry mouth, drowsiness, insomnia, sweating
Fluoxetine (Prozac)	10-80 mg/day	Insomnia or sedation, nausea, agitation, headaches
Paroxetine (Paxil)	20-50 mg/day	Insomnia or sedation, nausea, agitation, headaches
Sertraline (Zoloft)	50-200 mg/day	Insomnia or sedation, nausea, agitation, headaches
Venlafaxine (Effexor)	75-375 mg/day	↑ BP, agitation, sedation, insomnia, nausea
Antihistamines		
Fexofenadine (Allegra)	60 mg q12h	Minimal CNS and anticholinergic side effects
Antihyperlipidemics		
Atorvastatin (Lipitor)	10-80 mg/day	Headaches, dizziness, nausea, vomiting, diarrhea, myalgia, ↑ LFTs,

	10-80 mg/day	nausea, gas, diarrhea, abdominal cramps, pain, rash, itching
Pravastatin (Pravacol)	10-80 mg/day	Nausea, vomiting, diarrhea, constipation, headache, rash, itching, rhinitis
Rosuvastatin (Crestor)	5-40 mg/day	Same as atorvastatin
Simvastatin (Zocor)	5-80 mg/day	Same as atorvastatin
Antihypertensives		
Atenolol (Tenormin)	25-50 mg/day	Cold extremities, constipation, diarrhea, sweating, fatigue, dizziness, headache, nausea
Carvedilol (Coreg)	12.5-50 mg/day	Fatigue, Dizziness
Enalapril (Vasotec)	2.5-40 mg/day	Headaches, dizziness
Metoprolol (Lopressor)	100-400 mg/day	Decreased sexual function, drowsiness, insomnia, fatigue. weakness
Valsartan (Diovan)	80-160 mg/day	Rare
Antimigraine		
Rizatriptan (Maxalt)	5-30 mg/day	Drowsiness, dizziness, fatigue, tingling in extremities
Antipsychotics		
Aripiprazole (Abilify)	PO: 10-30 mg/day	Weight gain, headache, insomnia, vomiting
Olanzapine (Zyprexa)	PO: 5-20 mg/day	Drowsiness, agitation, insomnia, headache, nervousness, hostility, dizziness, rhinitis
Quetiapine (Seroquel)	PO: 300-800 mg/day	Headache, drowsiness, dizziness

continued

Common Drugs by Class (continued)

COMMON DRUGS	TYPICAL ADULT DOSES	COMMON SIDE EFFECTS
Antivirals		
Oseltamivir (Tamiflu)	75 mg bid × 5 days	Diarrhea, nausea, vomiting
Valacyclovir (Vatrex)	Shingles: 1 g tid × 7 days Genital herpes: 1 g bid × 3-10 days	Headaches, nausea
Bronchodilators		
Albuterol (ProAir, Proventil, Ventolin)	MDI: 2 puffs q4-6h prn Neb: 2.5 mg q4-6h prn	Headache, restlessness, nervousness, tremors, nausea, dizziness, throat irritation, heartburn
Fluticasone (Flovent)	MDI: 100-500 mcg q 12h Diskus: 100-500 g q 12h	Candidiasis, hoarseness, cough
Montelukast sodium (Singulair)	10 mg/day	Headache
Salmeterol/fluticasone (Advair)	Diskus: 1 puff q 12h	Headache, cough, hoarseness

Calcium Channel Blockers (essential hypertension)		
Amlodipine besylate (Norvasc)	2.5–10 mg/day	Peripheral edema, flushing, headaches
Diltiazem (Cardizem)	PO: 120–360 mg/day	Dizziness, drowsiness, peripheral edema, headache, fatigue, bradycardia
Cardiac Glycosides (CHF, arrhythmias)		
Amiodarone (Cordarone, Pacerone)	PO: Maintenance 200–600 mg/day	Blurry vision, constipation, headache, decreased appetite, nausea, vomiting
Digoxin (Lanoxin)	PO: maintenance 0.125–0.5 mg/day	Dizziness, headache, diarrhea, rash, visual disturbances
Corticosteroids (anti-inflammatory)		
Methylprednisolone (Medrol)	PO: 2–60 mg/day	Heartburn, anxiety, abdominal distension, sweating, acne, mood swings, facial flushing, diarrhea, constipation. delayed wound healing, ↑ appetite, weight gain, insomnia
Prednisone (Deltasone)	5–60 mg/day	Nausea, vomiting, appetite, weight gain, insomnia

continued

Common Drugs by Class (continued)

COMMON DRUGS	TYPICAL ADULT DOSES	COMMON SIDE EFFECTS
Diuretics		
Furosemide (Lasix)	HTN: 20-80 mg/day Edema: Up to 600 mg/day	Nausea, diarrhea, constipation, electrolyte disturbances, abdominal cramps
Hydrochlorothiazide (Mlcrozide)	HTN: 12.5-50 mg/day Edema: 25-100 mg/day	Potassium depletion, orthostatic hypotension
Opioid Analgesics		
Hydrocodone / acetaminophen (Lortab, Vicodan)	PO: 5-10 mg q 4h	Lethargy, hypotension, sweating, flushing, dizziness, drowsiness
Morphine (MS Contin)	PO: 10-30 mg/q 3-4h	Sedation, hypotension, sweating, flushing, constipation, dizziness, drowsiness, nausea, vomiting
Oxycodone (OxyContin)	PO: 5-20 mg/q4-6h	Drowsiness, dizziness, hypotension, anorexia
Sedatives		
Temazepam (Restoril)	7.5-30 mg/hs	Sedation, rebound insomnia, drowsiness, dizziness, confusion, euphoria
Zolpidem (Ambien)	5-10 mg/hs	Headaches
Thyroid		

Solution Compatibility Chart[28]

Intravenous Medication	D5W	D10W	D5/¼NS	D5/½NS	D5NS	NS	½NS	R	LR	D5LR
Acetazolamide	C	C	C	C	C	C	C	C	C	C
Acyclovir	C		C	C	C	C			C	
Aminophylline	C	C	C	C	C	C	C	C	C	C
Antithymocyte globulin	C	C	C	C	C	C	C			
Ascorbic acid	C	C	C	C	C	C	C	C	C	C
Aztreonam	C	C	C	C	C	C		C	C	C
Calcium chloride	C	C	C	C	C	C		C	C	C
Calcium gluconate	C	C			C	C			C	C
Cefazolin Na	C	C	C	C	C	C		C	C	C
Cefoperazone Na	C	C	C		C	C			C	C
Cefotaxime Na	C	C	C	C	C	C			C	
Cefotetan	C					C				
Cefoxitin Na	C	C	C	C	C	C		C	C	C
Ceftazidime	C	C	C	C	C	C		C	C	
Ceftizoxime Na	C	C	C	C	C	C		C	C	
Ceftriaxone Na	C	C		C		C				
Cefuroxime Na	C	C	C	C	C	C		C	C	
Cimetidine	C	C	C	C	C	C		C	C	C
Clindamycin	C	C		C	C	C			C	
Dexamethasone	C					C				
Dobutamine HCl	C	C		C	C	C	C		C	C
Dopamine HCl	C	C	C	C	C	C			C	C
Doxycycline	C					C		C		
Epinephrine	C	C	C	C	C	C		C	C	C
Famotidine	C	C				C			C	
Fentanyl	C					C				

Continued

Solution Compatibility (continued)

Intravenous Medication	D5W	D10W	D5/¼NS	D5/½NS	D5NS	NS	½NS	R	LR	D5LR
Folic acid	C					C				
Furosemide	C	C			C	C			C	C
Gentamicin	C	C				C		C	C	
Heparin Na	C		C	C	C	C	C	C		C
Hydrocortisone phosphate	C	C				C		C		
Hydrocortisone Na succinate	C	C	C	C	C	C	C	C	C	C
Hydromorphone HCl	C	C		C	C	C	C	C	C	C
Imipenem-Cilastatin	C⁴	C⁴	C⁴	C⁴	C⁴	C¹⁰				
Insulin (Regular)	Cᴾ	C		C		Cᴾ			C	
Isoproterenol	Cᴾ	C	C	C	C	C	Cᴾ		C	C
Kanamycin	C	C				C			C	
Labetalol	C		C		C	C		C	C	C
Lidocaine	Cᴾ			C	C	C	C		C	C
Magnesium sulfate	C					C			C	
Meperidine HCl	C	C	C	C	C	C	C	C	C	C
Meropenem	C¹	C¹	C¹		C¹	C⁴		C⁴	C⁴	C¹
Metoclopramide HCl	C			C					C	C
Morphine	C	C	C	C	C	C	C	C	C	C
Multivitamin	C	C				C	C		C	C
Nafcillin Na	C	C	C	C	C	C		C	C	
Nitroglycerin	C			C	C	C	C		C	C
Norepinephrine	Cᴾ					Cᴾ			C	
Ondansetron HCl	C			C	C	C				
Oxacillin Na	C	C			C	C			C	C
Pancuronium	C			C	C	C			C	
Papaverine	C	C	C	C	C	C	C	C		
Penicillin G, K	C	C	C	C	C	C	C	C	C	C

Intravenous Medication	D5W	D10W	D5/¼NS	D5/½NS	D5NS	NS	½NS	R	LR	D5LR
Pentobarbital Na	C	C	C	C	C	C	C	C	C	C
Piperacillin/ Tazobactam	C				C	C			C	
Potassium acetate	C	C				C			C	C
Potassium chloride	C	C	C	C	C	C	C	C	C	C
Potassium phosphate	C	C	C	C	C	C	C			
Prochlorperazine	C	C	C	C	C	C	C	C	C	C
Propranolol	C^P				C	C			C	
Pyridoxine HCl	C	C	C	C	C	C	C		C	C
Ranitidine	C	C	C		C	C			C	
Sodium acetate	C	C			C	C	C	C		C
Sodium bicarbonate	C	C	C	C						
Sodium chloride	C	C	C	C	C	C	C		C	C
Succinylcholine	C	C	C	C	C	C	C	C	C	C
Thiamine	C	C	C	C	C	C	C	C	C	C
Thiopental	C		C	C	C^6	C	C			
Trace metals	C	C			C	C			C	
Tranexamic acid	C	C	C	C	C	C	C		C	
Warfarin	C	C			C	C	C			C
Zidovudine	C^P					C				

FDA List of Generic Look-Alike Names and Recommended Revisions[17]

LOOK-ALIKE DRUG NAMES	SUGGESTED USE OF TALL MAN LETTERS
acetazolamide	aceta**ZOLAMIDE**
acetohexamide	aceta**HEXAMIDE**
bupropion	bu**PROP**ion
buspirone	bus**PIR**one
chlorpromazine	chlorpro**MAZINE**
chlorpropamide	chlorpro**PAMIDE**
clomiphene	clomi**PHENE**
clomipramine	clomi**PRAMINE**
cyclosporine	cyclo**SPORINE**
cycloserine	cyclo**SERINE**
daunorubicin	**DAUNO**rubicin
doxorubicin	**DOXO**rubicin
dimenhydrinate	dimenhy**DRINATE**
diphenhydramine	diphenhydr**AMINE**
dobutamine	**DOBUT**amine
dopamine	**DOP**amine
glipizide	glipi**ZIDE**
glyburide	gly**BURIDE**
hydralazine	hydr**ALAZINE**
hydroxyzine	hydr**OXY**zine
medroxyprogesterone	medroxy**PROGESTER**one
methylprednisolone	methyl**PREDNIS**olone
methyltestosterone	methyl**TESTOSTER**one
nicardipine	ni**CAR**dipine
nifedipine	**NIFE**dipine
prednisone	predni**SONE**
prednisolone	predniso**LONE**
sulfadiazine	sulf**ADIAZINE**
sulfisoxazole	sulfi**SOXAZOLE**
tolazamide	**TOLAZ**amide
tolbutamide	**TOLBUT**amide
Vinblastine	vin**BLAS**tine
Vincristine	vin**CRIS**tine

LABS

Labs

SEE ALSO

PROCEDURES

OBSTETRICS

PEDIATRICS

Routine Blood Chemistry[50]

TEST	NORMAL VALUES	SI UNITS
Glucose, fasting (FBS)		
Infant	40-90 mg/dL	2.2-5 mmol/L
Child <2 years	60-100 mg/dL	3.3-5.5 mmol/L
Child >2 years–adult	<110 mg/dL	<6.1 mmol/L
Hgb A1C		
Nondiabetic adult/child	4-5.9%	
Good diabetic control	<7%	
Fair diabetic control	8-9%	
Proteins		
Total	6.4-8.3 g/dL	64-83 g/L
Albumin	3.5-5 g/dL	35-50 g/L
Globulin	2.3-3.4 g/dL	23-34 g/L
BUN		
Child	5-18 mg/dL	
Adult	10-20 mg/dL	3.6-7.1 mmol/L
Creatinine		
Infant	0.2-0.4 mg/dL	
Child	0.3-0.7 mg/dL	
Adult	0.5-1.2 mg/dL	44-106 µmol/L
Bilirubin		
Total	0.3-1 mg/dL	5.1-17 µmol/L
Indirect	0.2-0.8 mg/dL	3.4-12 µmol/L
Direct	0.1-0.3 mg/dL	1.7-5.1 µmol/L
AST	0-35 units/L	0-0.58 µkat/L
ALP		
Child (9-15)	60-300 units/L	
Adult	30-120 units/L	0.5-2 µkat/L
ALT	4-36 international units/L @ 37° C	4-36 units/L
Electrolytes		
Calcium	9-10.5 mg/dL	2.25-2.75 mmol/L
Sodium	136-145 mEq/L	136-145 mmol/L
Potassium	3.5-5 mEq/L	3.5-5 mmol/L
Chloride	98-106 mEq/L	98-106 mmol/L
CO_2	23-30 mEq/L	23-30 mmol/L

ALT, alanine aminotransferase; **ALP**, alkaline phosphatase; **AST**, aspartate aminotransferase; **BUN**, blood urea nitrogen; **CO_2**, carbon dioxide; **FBS**, fasting blood sugar.

Labs

Complete Blood Cell Count with Differential[50]

TEST	NORMAL VALUES	SI UNITS
WBCs	5,000-10,000/mm³	5-10 × 10⁹/L
RBCs		
Male	4.7-6.1 × 10⁶/µL	4.7-6.1 × 10¹²/L
Female	4.2-5.4 × 10⁶/µL	4.2-5.4 × 10¹²/L
Hgb		
Child (1-6)	9.5-14 g/dL	
Child (6-18)	10-15.5 g/dL	
Adult Male	14-18 g/dL	8.7-11.2 mmol/L
Adult Female	12-16 g/dL	7.4-9.9 mmol/L
HCT		
Child (1-6)	30%-40%	
Child (6-18)	32%-44%	
Adult Male	42%-52%	0.42-0.52
Adult Female	37%-47%	0.37-0.47
MCV	82-95 fl	82-98 fl
MCH	27-31 pg	27-33 pg
MCHC	32%-36%	0.32-0.36
RDW	11%-14.5%	10.2%-14.5%
WBC diff		
Neutrophils	55%-70%	0.55-0.70
Lymphocytes	20%-40%	0.20-0.40
Monocytes	2%-8%	0.02-0.08
Eosinophils	1%-4%	0.01-0.04
Basophils	0.5%-1%	0.005-0.01
Plt count	150,000-400,000/mm³	150-400 × 10⁹/L
RBC Morphology		
(RBC smear)		
RBC	Normal size, shape, color	
RBC, WBC, Plt	Normal quantity	
WBC diff	Normal count	

iff, differential; **HCT,** hematocrit; **Hgb,** hemoglobin; **MCH,** mean orpuscular hemoglobin; **MCHC,** mean corpuscular hemoglobin oncentration; **MCV,** mean corpuscular volume; **Plt,** platelet; **RBC,** red blood cell; **RDW,** red blood cell distribution width ndex; **WBC,** white blood cell.

Arterial Blood Gases[50]

TEST	NORMAL VALUES	SI UNITS
pH	7.35-7.45	7.35-7.45
Pco_2	35-45 mm Hg	4.67-6 kPa
Po_2	80-100 mg Hg	10-13.33 kPa
HCO_3	21-28 mEq/L	
BXS	0%-2%	
O_2 sat	95%-100%	0.95-0.98 sat

Cardiac Enzymes[50]

TEST	NORMAL VALUES	SI UNITS
AST	0-35 units/L	0-0.58 μkat/L
CK		
Male	55-170 units/L	55-170 units/L
Female	30-135 units/L	30-135 units/L
LDH		
Child	60-170 units/L @ 30° C	
Adult	100-190 units/L @ 37° C	100-190 units/L
Myoglobin	<90 mcg/L	<90 mcg/L
Troponin I	<0.03 ng/mL	
Troponin T	<0.1 ng/mL	
CRP	<1 mg/dL	<10 mg/L

Coagulation Studies[50]

TEST	NORMAL VALUES	SI UNITS
PCT		
CEPI	89-193 sec	
CADP	64-120 sec	
PT	11-12.5 sec	11-12.5 sec
PTT	60-70 sec	60-70 sec
aPTT	30-40 sec	30-40 sec
Fibrinogen	200-400 mg/dL	2-4 g/L
Plasminogen	2.4-4.4 CTA units/mL	
Plt Count (thrombocyte count)	150,000-400,000/mm³	150-400 × 10⁹/L
MPV	7.4-10.4 fL	

aPTT, activated partial thromboplastin time; AST, aspartate aminotransferase; CADP, Collagen/adenosine–5'-diphosphate; CEPI, collagen/epinephrine; CK, Creatine Kinase; CRP, C-reactive protein; LDH, lactic dehydrogenase; MPV, mean platelet volume; PCT, platelet closure time; PT, prothrombin time; PTT, partial thromboplastin time.

Hepatic Function Panel[50]

TEST	NORMAL VALUES	SI UNITS
Albumin	3.5-5 g/dL	35-50 g/L
Bilirubin, total	0.3-1 mg/dL	5.1-17 μmol/L
Bilirubin, indirect	0.2-0.8 mg/dL	3.4-12 μmol/L
Bilirubin, direct	0.1-0.3 mg/dL	1.7-5.1 μmol/L
ALP		
Child (9-15)	60-300 units/L	
Adult	30-120 units/L	0.5-2 μkat/L
ALT	4-36 international units/L	4-36 units/L
AST	0-35 units/L	0-0.58 μkat/L
Protein, total	6.4-8.3 g/dL	64-83 g/L

Lipid Panel[50]

TEST	NORMAL VALUES	SI UNITS
Total cholesterol	<200 mg/dL (age dependent)	<5.20 mmol/L
HDL		
Male	>45 mg/dL	>0.75 mmol/L
Female	>55 mg/dL	>0.91 mmol/L
LDL		
Child	<110 mg/dL	
Adult	<130 mg/dL	
VLDL	7-32 mg/dL	
Triglycerides		
Male	40-160 mg/dL	0.45-1.81 mmol/L
Female	35-135 mg/dL	0.40-1.52 mmol/L

Thyroid Panel[50]

TEST	NORMAL VALUES	SI UNITS
T_4	5-12 mcg/dL	65-154 nmol/L
FT_4	0.8-2.8 ng/dL	10-36 pmol/L
Total T_3		
Adult (20-50)	70-205 ng/dL	1.2-3.4 nmol/L
Adult (>50 yrs)	40-180 ng/dL	0.6-2.8 nmol/L
TSH	0.3-5 uU/mL	0.3 U/L

ALP, alkaline phosphatase; **ALT**, alanine aminotransferase; **AST**, aspartate aminotransferase; **FT₄**, thyroxine, free; **HDL**, high-density lipoprotein; **LDL**, low-density lipoprotein; **T₃**, triiodothyronine; **T₄**, thyroxine; **TSH**, thyroid-stimulating hormone; **VLDL**, very-low-density lipoprotein.

Therapeutic Medication Levels[50]

TEST	THERAPEUTIC LEVEL	TOXIC LEVEL
Antiarrhythmics		
Lidocaine	1.5-5 mcg/mL	>5 mcg/mL
Procainamide	4-10 mcg/mL	>16 mcg/mL
Propranolol	50-100 ng/mL	>150 ng/mL
Quinidine	2-5 mcg/mL	>10 mcg/mL
Anticonvulsants		
Carbamazepine (Tegretol)	5-12 mcg/mL	>12 mcg/mL
Phenytoin (Dilantin)	10-20 mcg/mL	>30 mcg/mL
Phenobarbital	10-30 mcg/mL	>40 mcg/mL
Valproic acid	50-100 mcg/mL	>100 mcg/mL
Antipyretic		
Acetaminophen	Depends on use	>25 mcg/mL
Salicylate	100-250 mcg/mL	>300 mcg/mL
Bronchodilators		
Aminophylline	10-20 mcg/mL	>20 mcg/mL
Theophylline	10-20 mcg/mL	>20 mcg/mL
Digitalis preparations		
Digoxin	0.8-2.0 ng/mL	>2.4 ng/mL
Digitoxin	15-25 ng/mL	>25 ng/mL

Urinalysis[50]

TEST	NORMAL VALUES
Appearance	Clear
Color	Straw/amber
Odor	Aromatic
pH	4.6-8
Protein	Negative
Specific gravity	1.005-1.030
Glucose	Negative
Casts	None
WBCs	0-4
RBCs	<2

EMERGENCY/ECG

SEE ALSO

VITAL SIGNS/ASSESSMENT

OBSTETRICS

PEDIATRICS

BLS Guidelines for Cardiopulmonary Arrest—Adult[1, 4, 11]

CPR SEQUENCE	EXPLANATION AND GUIDELINE
Assess unresponsiveness	Attempt to arouse • If responsive CPR not needed • If unresponsive and no breathing or gasping detected, have someone activate EMS & get defibrillator*
Check pulse	Palpate carotid artery for up to 10 seconds • If pulse is present, begin breathing and recheck pulse every 2 minutes • If no pulse detected, deliver chest compressions
Chest compressions	Compressions should be given at a rate of 100/minute with depth of at least 2 inches. Push hard and fast for 30 compressions then open the airway
Open airway	If no trauma suspected, head tilt/chin lift position. If trauma suspected, jaw thrust only
Breathe	When airway open, give 2 breaths. Chest should rise and fall with each breath
Compression: ventilation ratio	30:2 (deliver 30 compressions, then 2 breaths)
Assess cardiac rhythm	When defibrillator is available, assess for shockable rhythm • If rhythm is not shockable, continue CPR and reassess rhythm every 5 cycles • If rhythm is shockable, defibrillate
Defibrillate	Deliver shock and resume CPR for 5 cycles then reassess rhythm

*Lone rescuer should perform 5 cycles of CPR before activating EMS

Pediatric Guidelines on pp. 158-159.

Cardiac Life Support Primary Survey[1,11]

Assess responsiveness ↓	Assess using AVPU: A=Alert; V=Responds to verbal stimuli; P=Responds to painful stimuli; U= unresponsive
RESPONSIVE	
Airway ↓	Determine responsiveness level
	Open, assess, and clear airway
Breathing ↓	Assess rate/quality of breathing
	If inadequate, assist ventilations with appropriate device and oxygen
Circulation ↓	Assess pulse rate and quality
	Assess perfusion
Defibrillation/ Disability	Assess need for defibrillator
	Obtain Glasgow coma score
	Perform Secondary Survey
UNRESPONSIVE	
Circulation ↓	If not breathing, assess pulse
	If no pulse, have someone activate EMS and obtain defibrillator
	Give 30 rapid chest compressions
Airway ↓	After 30 compressions, open the airway
Breathing ↓	Deliver 2 breaths; each breath should take about 1 second. Avoid excessive ventilation
Defibrillation	Apply AED, apply shock as needed, then resume CPR for 5 cycles ans reassess

Cardiac Life Support Secondary Survey: ABCDE[1,11]

Vital signs/ history	Obtain vital signs
	Attach Pulse oximeter, EKG and B/P monitor
	Obtain a focused history
Airway (advanced) ↓	Reassess airway.
	Reevaluate breathing.
	Perform endotracheal intubation if needed.
Breathing ↓	Assess ventilation.
	Confirm endotracheal tube placement.
	Provide positive-pressure ventilation with 100% O_2.
	Evaluate effectiveness of ventilations.
Circulation ↓	Establish peripheral vascular access.
	Attach ECG leads.
	Administer medications appropriate for cardiac rhythm and/or clinical situation.
Differential diagnosis	Consider possible causes of the arrest, rhythm, or situation.
Evaluation	Assess effectiveness of care.
	Troubleshoot as needed.
	Assess pain - begin appropriate pain management.
Family Presence	Facilitate family presence for invasive and resuscitative procedures.
	Explain what is being done to any family present

PQRST Mnemonic for Chest Pain Assessment[25]

	FACTOR	DESCRIPTION QUESTIONS
P	Provokes, palliates, precipitating factors	What provoked the pain? What makes the pain better? What makes the pain worse? Have you had this type of pain before? What were you doing when the pain occurred?
Q	Quality	What does the pain feel like? Is it burning? Crushing? Tearing? Sharp?
R	Region, radiation	Show me where the pain is. How large an area is involved? Does the pain radiate? If so, where?
S	Severity, associated symptoms	How severe is the pain? If you were to rate the pain on a scale from 0 to 10, with 10 being the most severe pain you can imagine, how would you rate your pain? What else did you feel besides the pain?
T	Time, temporal relations	When did the pain start? How long did it last? Does it come and go? Were you awakened by the pain? Is the pain always present?

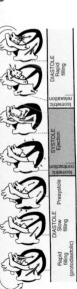

DIASTOLE Rapid filling (protodiastolic)	DIASTOLE Slow filling	Presystole	SYSTOLE Isometric contraction	SYSTOLE Ejection	Isometric relaxation	DIASTOLE Rapid filling

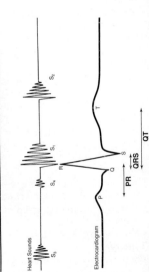

Normal Values
PR: 0.12–0.20 sec
QRS: 0.06–0.12 sec
QT: 0.32–0.44 sec

Heart Sounds — S₃, S₄, S₁, S₂

Electrocardiogram — P, Q, R, S, T

PR, QRS, QT

(Illustration from Jarvis C: Physical examination and health assessment, ed 6, Philadelphia, 2012, W.B. Saunders. Reprinted by permission.)

Systematic Evaluation of Cardiac Rhythms

Rate
- Bradycardia: <60/min
- Normal: 60-100/min
- Tachycardia: >100/min

Rhythm
- Is rhythm regular or irregular?

P Waves
- Are P waves present?
- Does one P wave appear before each QRS?

PR Interval
- Time it takes for impulse to spread from SA node through atrial muscle and AV node
- Measured from beginning of P wave to ventricular (QRS) complex
- Normal is 0.12-0.20 sec
- Is the interval prolonged? Shortened?

QRS Complex
- Time it takes for impulse to spread through right and left ventricles
- Measured from beginning of QRS to end of QRS
- Normal is 0.06-0.12 sec
- Are the QRS complexes normal shape and configuration?

QT Interval
- Time it takes for impulse to spread through ventricles and for repolarization to occur
- Measured from beginning of QRS to end of T wave
- Normal is 0.32-0.44 sec

ST Interval
- Is there deviation in the ST segment?
- ST elevation suggests infarction; ST depression suggests ischemia

EG Paper[2]

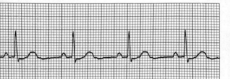

Horizontal lines measure time. Vertical lines measure amplitude or voltage.

Interpretation of Common Cardiac Rhythms[4]

Normal Sinus Rhythm

Rate	60-100
Rhythm	Regular
P waves	Similar; 1:1 with QRS
PR	0.12-0.20 sec; constant
QRS	≤0.1 sec

Sinus Bradycardia

Rate	<60
Rhythm	Regular
P waves	Similar; 1:1 with QRS
PR	0.12-0.20 sec; constant
QRS	≤0.1 sec

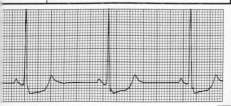

Sinus Tachycardia

Rate	101-180
Rhythm	Regular
P waves	Similar; 1:1 with QRS; at very fast rates, P wave looks like T wave
PR	0.12-0.20 sec; constant
QRS	≤0.1 sec

Sinus Arrhythmia

Rate	60-100
Rhythm	Irregular; often associated with breathing
P waves	Similar; 1:1 with QRS
PR	0.12-0.20 sec; constant
QRS	≤0.1 sec

Premature Atrial Contraction

Rate	Variable
Rhythm	Regular with premature beats
P waves	Premature; 1:1 with QRS
PR	Dependent on prematurity of the beat
QRS	Usually <0.1 sec, but may be wide

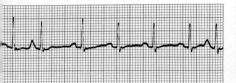

Supraventricular Tachycardia

Rate	150-250
Rhythm	Regular
P waves	Usually obscure but 1:1 with QRS
PR	0.12-0.20 sec when present
QRS	Usually <0.1 sec

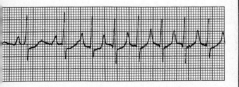

Atrial Tachycardia

Rate	150-250
Rhythm	Regular
P waves	P waves appear different; may be difficult to distinguish P waves from T waves
PR	May be shorter or longer than normal; may be hard to measure
QRS	Usually ≤0.1 sec

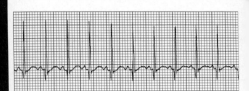

Atrial Flutter

Rate	Atrial 250-450; ventricular rate variable
Rhythm	Atrial regular; ventricular may be regular or irregular
P waves	No P waves. Flutter (sawtooth-shaped) waves observed
PR	Not measurable
QRS	Usually <0.1 sec

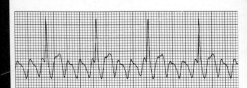

Atrial Fibrillation

Rate	Atrial 400-600; ventricular variable
Rhythm	Ventricular irregular
P waves	No P wave; fibrillatory waves may be present; erratic, wavy baseline
PR	Not measurable
QRS	Usually <0.1 sec

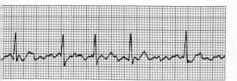

Premature Ventricular Contraction

Rate	60-100
Rhythm	Regular with PVCs
P waves	Absent; may appear after QRS complex
PR	None
QRS	>0.12 sec; wide and bizarre

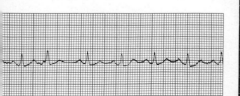

Ventricular Tachycardia

Rate	150-300, typically 200-250
Rhythm	May be regular or irregular
P waves	None
PR	None
QRS	>0.12 sec

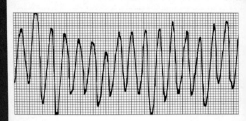

Asystole

Rate	None
Rhythm	None
P waves	None ("P-wave" asystole)
PR	None
QRS	Absent

Ventricular Fibrillation	
Rate	Cannot be determined—no discernible waves or complexes to measure
Rhythm	Rapid and chaotic—no pattern
P waves	None
PR	None
QRS	Not discernible

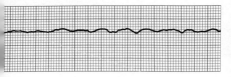

ne ventricular fibrillation.

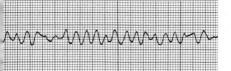

oarse ventricular fibrillation.

First-Degree AV Block

Rate	Usually normal 60-100
Rhythm	Regular
P waves	Similar, 1:1 with QRS
PR	Prolonged (>0.20 sec) but constant
QRS	Usually ≤0.10 sec

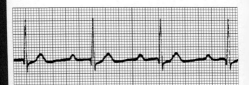

Second-Degree AV Block, Type I

Rate	Atrial > ventricular
Rhythm	Atrial regular; ventricular irregular
P waves	Similar, more P waves than QRS
PR	Lengthens with each cycle until a P wave appears without a QRS
QRS	Usually ≤0.10 sec; QRS cycle is periodically dropped

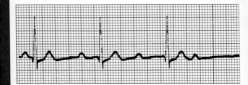

Second-Degree AV Block, Type II

Rate	Atrial > ventricular
Rhythm	Atrial regular; ventricular rhythm irregular
P waves	Similar, more P waves than QRS
PR	May be normal or prolonged; remains constant
QRS	Usually ≥0.10 sec; QRS cycle may be absent after P waves

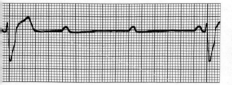

Third-Degree AV Block

Rate	Atrial > ventricular; usually slow ventricular rate between 30-60
Rhythm	Atrial and ventricular; no relationship between the two
P waves	Similar; more P waves than QRS
PR	None; atria and ventricles beat independently of each other
QRS	May be narrow or wide depending on level of the block

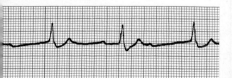

omplete AV block with a junctional escape
acemaker (QRS = 0.08-0.10 sec).

Electrocardiograph Lead Placement[40]

ECG lead placement. **A**, Lead placement for limb leads I, II, and III. **B**, Limb leads aV$_R$, aV$_L$, aV$_F$. **C**, Lead placement for chest leads V$_1$-V$_6$.

Localizing Ischemia, Injury, or Infarct with 12-Lead ECG[9]	
Leads with Changes	**Affected Area of Heart**
I, aVL, V$_5$, V$_6$	Lateral wall ischemia, injury, or infarct
II, III, aVF	Inferior wall ischemia, injury, or infarct
V$_1$, V$_2$	Septal wall ischemia, injury, or infarct
V$_3$, V$_4$	Anterior wall ischemia, injury, or infarct

Relief of Foreign-Body Airway Obstruction[10,11]

Adult—(8 years of age and older)

1. Ask "Are you choking? Can you speak?"
2. If victim cannot speak or exhibits stridor, then give abdominal thrusts/Heimlich maneuver (see below) or chest thrusts for pregnant or obese victims.
3. Repeat thrusts until effective or victim becomes unresponsive.

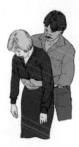

If victim becomes unresponsive:

4. Activate the EMS system.
5. Lower patient to the ground and begin CPR with 30 chest compressions.
6. Open airway, check for and remove any visible foreign body and then give 2 rescue breaths.
7. Repeat steps 5 and 6 until effective.*

*If victim is breathing or resumes effective breathing, place in the recovery position.

Guidelines for Stroke Management[11]
Recognition of Stroke Symptoms,
Activate EMS

Prehospital Care

- Support ABC's; oxygen as needed
- Prehospital stroke assessment
- Establish time of onset of symptoms
- Transport to stroke center, alert hospital
- Check glucose if possible

ED Arrival (within first 10 minutes of ED arrival)

- Assess airway, breathing, circulation
- Oxygen, IV access, blood samples, including glucose
- Neurologic screening assessment
- Activate Stroke Team
- Order emergent CT scan
- Obtain 12 lead ECG

Stroke Team (within 25 minutes of ED arrival)

- Review history, establish onset of symptoms
- Neurologic examination (NIH Stroke Scale or Canadian Neurologic Scale)

CT Scan (within 45 minutes of ED arrival)

- If evidence of hemorrhage, consult with neurologist/neurosurgeon
- If no evidence of hemorrhage, consider fibrinolytic therapy. If not candidate for fibrinolytic therapy, administer aspirin, and admit to stroke unit.

Fibrinolytic Therapy (within 60 minutes of ED arrival)

- If candidate, initiate rtPA (No anticoagulants/antiplatelets for 24 hrs)
- Admit to stroke unit or ICU.

Care of the Patient During a Seizure[53]

Note: Mainlining an open airway and patient safety are Priority 1)

During Seizure

- Call for help and stay with patient.
- Do NOT restrain the patient.
- Time the seizure.
- Place something soft under the head.
- Turn patient on side.
- Remove glasses and loosen tight clothing.
- Do NOT place anything between teeth.
- Do NOT attempt to remove dentures.
- Monitor the duration of the seizure and the type of movement.

After Seizure

- Keep patient on side to allow saliva to drain; suction if needed.
- Obtain vital signs and perform neurologic checks as needed.
- Reorient patient, and allow to rest.
- Do NOT offer food or drink until fully awake.
- Notify provider.
- Record all observations during and after the seizure.
  - document time and length of seizure
  - Document occurrence of an aura (if aura occurred, note the sequence of behaviors)
  - document any injuries during seizure and how the injuries were treated.
  - document post seizure events such as time consciousness regained and reorientation of patient.

Indication of Neurologic Injury — Posturing[40]

	DECORTICATE	DECEREBRATE
Lesion Location	Cerebral hemisphere	Midbrain or upper brainstem
Clinical Signs	• Flexion posturing • Unilateral or bilateral flexion of arms, wrists, and fingers • Shoulder abduction and flexion • Extension, internal rotation, and plantar flexion of the feet	• Teeth clenched • All four extremities in rigid extension, with hyperpronation of forearms • Legs extended • Plantar flexion of the feet

TRAUMA

Primary and Secondary Assessment of the Trauma Patient

- Primary Assessment
  - **A**—Airway
  - **B**—Breathing
  - **C**—Circulation
  - **D**—Disability (neurologic status)
- Secondary Assessment
  - **E**—Expose (remove clothing; keep patient warm)
  - **F**—Full set of vital signs
  - **G**—Give comfort measures
  - **H**—History/Head-to-toe assessment
  - **I**—Inspect posterior surfaces

Trauma Score

AREA OF MEASUREMENT	FINDINGS	SCORE
Glasgow Coma Scale*	13-15	4
	9-12	3
	6-8	2
	4-5	1
	0-3	0
Systolic blood pressure	>89 mm Hg	4
	76-89 mm Hg	3
	50-75 mm Hg	2
	1-49 mm Hg	1
	0	0
Respiratory rate (patient-initiated ventilations)	10-29/min	4
	>29/min	3
	6-9/min	2
	1-5/min	1
	0	0
Total possible points		0-12[†]

*See Glasgow Coma Scale on p. 39.
†The lower the score the more severe the trauma.

Burn Assessment and Management

Burn Assessment

- Depth of burn
- Partial thickness (superficial = 1st degree; deep = 2nd degree)
- Full thickness = 3rd degree
- Extent of burn: estimate percent body surface area (BSA) affected using rule o nines (below)
- Location of burn
- Presence of other injuries (i.e., pulmonary, trauma)

Emergent Management

- Airway management (intubate if necessary)
- Fluid resuscitation formula and infusion schedule (first 24 hours)

  % BSA × Body weight (kg) × 4 mL
  Lactated Ringers

  50% given 1st 8 hours
  25% given 2nd 8 hours
  25% given 3rd 8 hours

Rule of Nines[27]

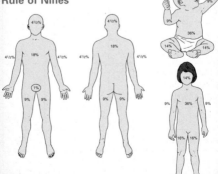

Emergency Cardiac Drugs—Quick List

MEDICATION	ADULT DOSAGE/ADMINISTRATION	USE
Adenosine	6 mg rapid IVP, then 12 mg IV q1-2min × 2 prn. Half-life <10 sec; give at closest IV port, follow with IV flush	Symptomatic SVT; monomorphic VTAC
Alteplase (tPA)	15 mg IV bolus followed by infusion 0.75 mg/kg over next 20 minutes, followed by infusion 0.5 mg/kg over next 60 minutes	Fibrinolytic; treatment of acute developing myocardial infarction
Amiodarone	Rapid infusion 150-300 mg IV over 10 min; follow with 1 mg/min infusion	Persistent or recurrent VF or pulseless VT
Atropine	0.5-1.0 mg IV q3-5min prn max 0.03-0.04 mg/kg Can be given through ET tube 2-2.5 times normal IV dose	Symptomatic bradycardia, asystole
Dobutamine	Continuous IV infusion; usual dose is 2-20 mcg/kg/min IV, based on patient response	Short-term management of cardiac decompensation resulting from depressed contractility

Continued

Emergency Cardiac Drugs (continued)

Dopamine	Continuous IV infusion: dose range: 5-20 mcg/kg/min; begin infusion at 5 mcg/kg/min; increase infusion rate according to BP and other clinical responses	Hemodynamically significant hypotension in the absence of hypovolemia
Epinephrine	0.1-1.0 mg IV, repeat q5min prn Can also be given through ET tube 2-2.5 times normal IV dose	Cardiac arrest, anaphylaxis, bradycardia
Isoproterenol	IV 0.02-0.06, then 0.01-0.2 mcg/min	Heart block, ventricular dysrhythmias
Lidocaine	1.5 mg/kg to total of 3 mg/kg IV; follow by continuous infusion 1-4 mg/min Can be given through ET tube 2-2.5 times normal IV dose	VT, VF, PVCs
Magnesium	1-2 g IVP	Torsades de pointes, or when dysrhythmia caused by hypomagnesium
Nitroglycerin	SL 0.4 mg IV infusion: initiate at 5 mcg/min, increase every 3-5 min until pain free, BP >90, or maximal dose to 20 mcg/min	Ischemic chest pain; improves coronary perfusion

Norepinephrine	IV infusion: Initiate infusion at 2 mcg/min and titrate to desired BP; usual range = 2-12 mcg/min	Short-term use for hypotension or shock
Procainamide	20-30 mg/min, max = 17 mg/kg or 500 mg	Recurrent VF, VT, PVCs
Propranolol HCl	IVP: 0.5-3 mg. Give slowly 1 mg/min; may repeat dose after 2 min	Control of hypertension and suppression of rapid-rate cardiac dysrhythmias
Reteplase	10 units IV bolus over 2 min; after 10 min, administer 2nd 10 units IV bolus over 2 min	Fibrinolytic; treatment of acute developing myocardial infarction
Streptokinase	1.5 million international units over 1 hr infusion	Fibrinolytic; treatment of acute developing myocardial infarction
Vasopressin	Dilute with D5W Cardiac arrest: 40 units IV x 1 Other: 0.5 milliunit/kg/hr Maximum: 10 miliunits/kg/hr	Alternative to epinephrine for VF or pulseless VT; short-term use for hypotension or shock
Verapamil	10-15 mg slow IVP (over 2 min), repeat in 30 min	SVT or atrial fib/flutter

Other Common Emergency Drugs—Quick List

MEDICATION	ADULT DOSAGE/ADMINISTRATION	USE
Albuterol	Neb: 2.5-5.0 mg in 2 mL q4h; inhaler: 1-2 puffs q4h. Neb can be given as continuous with 2-3 doses over 1 hr	Acute bronchospasm
Dexamethasone	PO/IM/IV: 0.75-9 mg/day in divided doses	Asthma, allergic reactions, spinal injury
Diazepam	5-10 mg IV q10-15min prn, max 20 mg. Administer slow IVP	Seizures
Heparin	35-70 units/kg IV bolus followed by 15-18 units/kg/hr continuous infusion. Subcutaneous injection: 5000 units q8-12h	Anticoagulation
Naloxone	0.2-2 mg IV; repeat q2-3min if necessary. Can also be given via ET tube	Reversal of narcotic effects, altered LOC
Mannitol	0.5-1.0 g/kg IV over 20 min, repeat if needed after 5 min	Cerebral edema, increased ICP

OBSTETRICS

Obstetrics

Signs of Pregnancy[42]

TIME OF OCCURRENCE (GESTATIONAL AGE)	SIGN	OTHER POSSIBLE CAUSES
Presumptive Signs		
3-4 wk	Breast changes	Premenstrual changes, oral contraceptives
4 wk	Amenorrhea	Stress, vigorous exercise, early menopause, endocrine problems, malnutrition
4-14 wk	Nausea, vomiting	GI upset, food poisoning
6-12 wk	Urinary frequency	Infection, pelvic tumors
12 wk	Fatigue	Stress, illness
16-20 wk	Quickening	Gas, peristalsis
Probable Signs		
5 wk	Softening of cervix (Goodell's sign)	Pelvic congestion
6-8 wk	Bluish tinge of vulva/vagina (Chadwick's sign)	Pelvic congestion
6-12 wk	Softening of cervical isthmus (Hegar's sign)	Pelvic congestion
4-12 wk	Positive pregnancy test (serum)	Hydatidiform mole, choriocarcinoma

6-12 wk	Positive pregnancy test (urine)	Pelvic infection, tumor
16 wk	Braxton Hicks contractions	Myomas, other tumors
16-28 wk	Ballottement	Tumors, cervical polyps
Positive Signs		
5-6 wk	Visualization of fetus by real-time ultrasound examination	No other causes
6 wk	Fetal heart tones detected by ultrasound examination	
8-17 wk	Fetal heart tones detected by Doppler ultrasound stethoscope	
16 wk	Visualization of fetus by x-ray study	
17-19 wk	Fetal heart tones detected by fetal stethoscope	
19-22 wk	Fetal movements palpated	
Late pregnancy	Fetal movements visible	

DELIVERY DATE CALCULATIONS

Nägele's Rule

	Worksheet	Example
First day of patient's last period	_____	Jan 14, 2016
Add 7 days	_____	Jan 21, 2016
Subtract 3 months	_____	Oct 21, 2015
Add 1 year	_____	*Oct 21, 2016 EDB

(*This calculated date is the estimated date of birth.)

GRAVIDITY/PARITY (GTPAL)[43,58]

G = gravidity (number of pregnancies)
T = number of term births (specify term subtype)
  Early term (37 0/7-38 6/7 wks)
  Full term (39 0/7-40 6/7 wks)
  Late term (41 0/7-41 6/7 wks)
  Post term (42 0/7 wks or greater)
P = number of preterm births (20 0/7-36 6/7 weeks)
A = number of abortions/miscarriages (<20 weeks)
L = number of living children

Eg: 31112 GTPAL = 3 pregnancies, 1 term birth, 1 preterm birth, 1 abortion & 2 living children

Immunizations During Pregnancy[20]

Vaccine	Recommendations
Hepatitis A and B	Yes if at risk for disease
HPV	No, under study
Influenza IIV	Yes
Influenza LAIV	No
MMR	No
Meningococcal	If exposed and indicated
Pneumococcal	If exposed and indicated
Tdap	Yes ideally between 27-36 wks
Varicella	No

*Consult www.cdc.gov/vaccines for additional information.

Vital Signs[42]

Vital Signs	Expected Change
Temperature	Slight ↑
Pulse	↑ 10-15 beats/min
Respirations	Unchanged or slight ↑
BP*	↓ 2nd trimester, returns to prepregnancy levels in 3rd trimester
MAP	Slight ↑

Very positional—take in same arm, same position, and record arm and position with reading

Calculation of Mean Arterial Pressure*[42]

Formula:

$$\frac{(systolic) + 2(diastolic)}{3} = MAP$$

Example: BP: 106/70

$$\frac{(106) + 2(70)}{3} =$$

$$\frac{106 + 140}{3} =$$

$$\frac{246}{3} = \textbf{82 mm Hg}$$

*Calculating MAP can increase the validity of blood pressure findings in pregnant women.

Body Systems[42]

SYSTEM	ANATOMY & PHYSIOLOGY CHANGES	MANIFESTATIONS
Reproductive	Uterus enlarges, changes shape and position	Fundal height palpable after 12-14 weeks
	↑ Uterine contractility & blood flow	Irregular painless contractions
	Cervix softens, glands proliferate	Soft tip, velvety appearance
	Fetus develops	Abdomen enlarges
		Fetal movement at 14-18 weeks
	Vaginal mucosa thickens	Leukorrhea (white or grey discharge)
	Vaginal secretions pH more acidic	↑ Susceptibility for yeast infection
	Vagina hypertrophies, vault lengthens	Palpable
	↑ Vaginal vascularity	Mucosa is violet-blue, ↑ Sexual arousal
Breasts	↑ Estrogen and progesterone	Breast fullness, sensitivity, heaviness
		↑ Pigment in nipples & areola
	↑ Vascularity of breast vessels	Bluish network of vessels visible
	Growth of mammary glands	Progressive breast enlargement
	↑ Luteal hormones promote rise of lactiferous ducts	Breasts feel coarser
	Glandular tissue replaces soft breast tissue	Breasts feel softer & looser

Cardiovascular	Heart enlarges, elevates, and rotates	Split S_1 and S_2, S_3 common
	↑ Upward volume, ↑ Cardiac output	Pulmonic murmurs
	↑ Venous pressure	Edema
	↓ Blood to legs	Varicosities, hemorrhoids
Respiratory	↑ Metabolic rate/↑ Tidal volume/↑ Oxygen consumption	Fatigue, heat intolerance
		Dyspnea at rest
	Chest expands/ribs flare out/diaphragm displaced	Nasal stuffiness, nose bleeds, mild URIs, earaches, fullness in ear
	↑ Vascularity upper respiratory tract	
Renal	Compressed bladder/ureters	UTI susceptibility
	Slowed urine flow rate and urine stagnation	Urinary urgency and frequency
	Impaired glucose reabsorption	Glycosuria
Skin	Hyperpigmentation	Darkened nipples, areola, axillae, vulva, chloasma, linea nigra
	Separation of collagen tissue	Stretch marks
	↑ Estrogen	Vascular spiders, palmar erythema
	↑ Blood flow to skin	↑ Perspiration, ↑ Nail growth, gum hypertrophy

continued

Body Systems (continued)

SYSTEM	ANATOMY & PHYSIOLOGY CHANGES	MANIFESTATIONS
Musculoskeletal	↑ Weight	Gait alteration, "waddle"
	Expanding abdomen	Belly button protrudes
	Pelvis tilt	Aching, numbness in arms
	↑ Spinal curve	Backaches
	Softening connective tissue and separation of pubis symphysis	Pain and difficulty in walking
Neurologic	Compression of pelvic nerves	Numbness in legs
	Edema of peripheral nerves	Pain, burning in hands, headache
GI system	↑ hCG	Morning sickness
	↑ Metabolism	↑ Appetite, food cravings
	Reverse peristalsis	Heartburn
	↓ Peristalsis	Constipation
Endocrine	↑ Thyroid hormone	Possible enlargement of thyroid
	Increased insulin production	Hypoglycemia
	Increased insulin resistance	Possible pregestational diabetes
General		Weight gain 25 lb on average

Laboratory Values[42]

TESTS	PREGNANT
Complete blood cell (CBC) count	
Hemoglobin	>11 g/dL*
Hematocrit	>33%*
Red blood cell (RBC) volume	Decreased
RBC count	20-30% increase
White blood cell (WBC) count	Normal to slight increase
Neutrophils	Slight increase
Lymphocytes	Normal to slight decrease
Coagulation	
prothrombin time (PT)	Slight ↓
partial thromboplastin time (PTT)	Slight ↓, and further ↓ during 2nd and 3rd stages of labor
Platelets	Rapid ↑ 3-5 days after birth and then gradual return to normal
Glucose, Blood fasting	Slight decrease
Serum Proteins	
Total	Slight decrease
Albumin	Slight increase
Globulin	Slight increase
Blood Urea Nitrogen (BUN)	Decreases
Creatinine	Decreases
Arterial Blood gases	
pH	Slight increase
PCO_2	Decreased
PO_2	Increased
HCO_3	Decreased

At sea level. Permanent residents of higher levels (e.g., Denver) require higher levels of hemoglobin.
Normal values can be found under Labs tab pp-76-60

Distinguishing True from False Labor[42]

True Labor

Contractions

- Occur regularly, become stronger, last longer, and occur closer together
- Become more intense with walking
- Usually felt in lower back, radiating to lower abdomen
- Continue despite use of comfort measures

Cervix (by vaginal examination)

- Progressive change (softening, effacement, dilation signaled by bloody show)
- Moves to anterior position

Fetus

- Presenting part usually becomes engaged in the pelvis, results in easier breathing. At the same time, presenting part presses downward and compresses bladder, causing urinary frequency

False Labor

Contractions

- Occur irregularly or temporarily regular
- Often stops with walking
- Felt in back or abdomen above navel
- Often stopped with comfort measures

Cervix (by vaginal examination)

- May be soft; no significant change in effacement
- No dilation or evidence of bloody show
- Often in a posterior position

Fetus

- Presenting part usually not engaged

Factors Affecting Labor (5 Ps)[42]

FACTOR	EXAMPLES
Passenger (fetus and placenta)	Size of head Fetal presentation Fetal lie Fetal attitude Fetal position
Passageway (birth canal)	Bony pelvis Pelvic floor Cervix
Powers (contractions)	Effacement/dilation cervix Contraction force/length
Position (mother's)	Comfort
Psychologic (maternal response)	Pain Anxiety Preparation/support

Labor Stages[42]

STAGE	SIGNS
I	From onset of contractions to full effacement and dilation of cervix *Latent:* 0–3 cm dilation *Active:* 4–7 cm dilation *Transition:* 8–10 cm dilation
II	From full cervical dilation to birth of baby *Latent:* rest and calm between contractions *Active pushing (descent):* urge to bear down and active bearing-down behaviors
III	From birth of baby to expulsion of placenta Placental separation & expulsion (10-15 min) Placental expulsion
IV	First 1 to 2 hrs after birth Physiological recovery from birth process

Fetal Vertex Presentations[42]

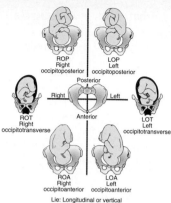

ROP
Right occipitoposterior

LOP
Left occipitoposterior

Posterior

Right — Left

Anterior

ROT
Right occipitotransverse

LOT
Left occipitotransverse

ROA
Right occipitoanterior

LOA
Left occipitoanterior

Lie: Longitudinal or vertical
Presentation: Vertex
Reference point: Occiput
Attitude: General flexion

Other Fetal Presentations[42]

A Frank breech

Lie: Longitudinal or vertical
Presentation: Breech (incomplete)
Presenting part: Sacrum
Attitude: Flexion, except for legs at knees

B Single footling breech

Lie: Longitudinal or vertical
Presentation: Breech (incomplete)
Presenting part: Sacrum
Attitude: Flexion, except for one leg extended at hip and knee

C Complete breech

Lie: Longitudinal or vertical
Presentation: Breech (sacrum and feet presenting)
Presenting part: Sacrum (with feet)
Attitude: General flexion

D Shoulder presentation

Lie: Transverse or horizontal
Presentation: Shoulder
Presenting part: Scapula
Attitude: Flexion

Fetal Station[42]

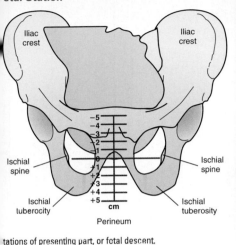

stations of presenting part, or fetal descent.

Dilation and Effacement of Cervix[42]

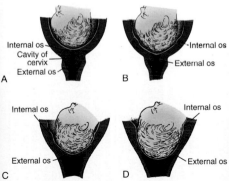

A, Before Labor; **B,** early effacement;
C, complete effacement; **D,** complete dilation

Interventions for Emergencies[43]

SIGNS	INTERVENTIONS*
Nonreassuring FHR pattern • FHR <110 bpm for >10 min† • FHR >160 bpm for >10 min in term pregnancy§ • Irregular FHR, abnormal sinus rhythm • Persistent ↓ in baseline FHR variability without any identified cause • Late, severe variable, prolonged deceleration patterns • Absence of FHR	Change woman to maternal position Discontinue oxytocin infusion Increase IV fluid rate or start IV Administer O_2 8-10 L/min by mask Check maternal temperature Assist with amnioinfusion if ordered Stimulate fetal scalp or use acoustic stimulation
Inadequate uterine relaxation • Intrauterine pressure >75 mm Hg • Contractions consistently lasting >90 sec • Contraction interval <2 min	Change woman to maternal position Discontinue oxytocin infusion Increase IV fluid rate or start IV Administer O_2 8-10 L/min by mask Palpate and evaluate contractions Give tocolytics (terbutaline), as ordered
Vaginal bleeding • Vaginal bleeding (in excess of that expected) • Continuous vaginal bleeding with FHR changes • Pain; may or may not be present	Anticipate emergency (stat) cesarean birth DO NOT PERFORM VAGINAL EXAM

Infection • Foul-smelling amniotic fluid • Maternal temperature >38° C in presence of adequate hydration • FHR >160 bpm† or >10 min	Institute cooling measures for woman Start an IV line if not in place Collect catheterized urine specimen and amniotic fluid sample for lab analysis

Prolapse of cord
• Fetal bradycardia with variable deceleration during uterine contraction
• Woman reports feeling cord after membrane rupture
• Cord lies alongside or below presenting part of fetus; can be seen or felt in or protruding from the vagina
• Major predisposing factors are the following:
  • ROM with a gush
  • Loose fit of presenting part in lower uterine segment
  • Presenting part not yet engaged
  • Breech presentation
	Call for assistance
	Glove hand; insert two fingers into vagina to cervix; exert upward pressure against presenting part to relieve cord compression
	Place rolled towel under woman's hips
	Place woman in modified Sims', extreme Trendelenburg, or knee-chest position
	Administer O_2 at 8-10 L/min by mask until birth
	Increase IV fluid rate or start IV
	Monitor FHR
	DO NOT replace cord into cervix; wrap any protruding cord loosely in sterile towel saturated with warm normal saline
	Prepare for immediate birth (vaginal or cesarean)

bpm, beats per minute; **FHR**, fetal heart rate; **IV**, intravenous; **stat**, immediately; **ROM**, rupture of membranes.

*Notify primary health care provider in all identified situations.

†Practice is to intervene within 2 to 30 minutes of FHR <110 bpm.

§Nonreassuring sign when associated with late decelerations or absence of variability, especially of >180 bpm.

123

Fetal Heart Rate Assessment[46]

1. What is the baseline FHR?
   __Beats per minute (bpm)

   Check one of the following as observed
   on the monitor strip:
   __Average baseline FHR (normal range of
   110-160 bpm)
   __Tachycardia (>160 bpm)
   __Bradycardia (<110 bpm)

2. What is the baseline variability?
   __Absent (range undetectable)
   __Minimal (> undetectable to ≤5 bpm)
   __Moderate (6-25 bpm)
   __Marked (>25 bpm)

3. Are there any periodic (or episodic) changes
   in the FHR?
   __Accelerations with fetal movement
   __Accelerations with uterine compression
   __Early decelerations (head compression)
   __Late decelerations (uteroplacental
   insufficiency)
   __Variable decelerations (cord
   compression)
   ____Reassuring (<30-45 sec, abrupt return
   to baseline, normal baseline rate,
   moderate variability)
   ____Nonreassuring (>60 sec, slow return
   to baseline, increasing baseline rate,
   absence of variability)
   ____Prolonged deceleration (>15 bpm
   below baseline, >2 min to <10 min)

4. What is the uterine activity/uterine contrac-
   tion (UC) pattern?
   __Frequency (onset to onset of UC)
   __Duration (beginning to end of
   contraction)
   __Intensity in mm Hg
   __Resting time ≥30 sec
   __Resting tone (<15 mm Hg pressure)

NEWBORN

APGAR Scoring System (Range = 0-10)

Category	0	1	2
Heart rate (bpm)	Absent	<100	100
Respirations	Absent	Slow, irregular	Good, crying
Muscle tone	Limp	Some flexion	Active motion
Reflex irritability (catheter in nares, tactile stimulation)	No response	Grimace	Cough, sneeze, cry
Color	Blue or pale	Pink body with blue extremities	Completely pink

Vital Signs (First 12 Hours of Life)[42]

Heart rate (awake): 100-160 bpm
Respiratory rate: 30-60 breaths/min

Systolic blood pressure: 60-80 mm Hg
Diastolic blood pressure: 40-50 mm Hg

Initial Physical Assessment by Body System[a]

CNS
- [ ] Moves extremities, muscle tone good
- [ ] Suck, rooting, Moro response, grasp reflexes good
- [ ] Anterior fontanel soft and flat

CV
- [ ] Heart rate strong and regular
- [ ] No murmurs heard
- [ ] Pulses strong and equal bilaterally

RESP
- [ ] Lungs clear to auscultation bilaterally
- [ ] No retractions or nasal flaring
- [ ] Respiratory rate, 30-60 breaths/min
- [ ] Chest expansion symmetric
- [ ] No upper airway congestion

GU
- [ ] Male: urethral opening at tip of penis; testes descended bilaterally
- [ ] Female: vaginal opening apparent

GI
- [ ] Abdomen soft, no distention
- [ ] Cord attached and clamped
- [ ] Anus appears patent

ENT
- [ ] Eyes clear
- [ ] Palates intact
- [ ] Nares patent

SKIN
Color [ ] Pink   [ ] Acrocyanotic
- [ ] No lesions or abrasions
- [ ] No peeling
- [ ] Birthmarks_____
- [ ] Caput and molding
- [ ] Vacuum "cap"
- [ ] Forceps marks
- [ ] Other

Comments_____

Abruptio Placenta/Placenta Previa Findings[42]

	Abruptio Placenta			Placenta Previa
	Grade 1 Mild Separation (10%–20%)	**Grade 2** Moderate Separation (20%–50%)	**Grade 3** Severe Separation (>50%)	
General findings				
Bleeding, external, vaginal	Minimal	Absent or moderate	Absent to moderate	Minimal to severe
Total amount of blood loss	<500 mL	1000–1500 mL	>1500 mL	Varies
Color of blood	Dark red	Dark red	Dark red	Bright red
Shock	Rare: none	Mild	Common, often sudden	Uncommon
Coagulopathy	Rare: none	Occasional DIC	Frequent DIC	None
Uterine tonicity	Normal	Increased	Tetanic	Normal
Tenderness (pain)	Usually absent	Present	Agonizing pain	Absent
Ultrasonographic findings				
Location of placenta	Normal, upper uterine segment	Normal, upper uterine segment	Normal, upper uterine segment	Abnormal, lower uterine segment
Station of presenting part	Variable to engaged	Variable to engaged	Variable to engaged	High, not engaged
Fetal position	Usual variations	Usual variations	Usual variations	Commonly transverse, breech, or oblique

Diagnostic Criteria for Preeclampsia and Preeclampsia with Severe Features[7]

Component	Preeclampsia	Severe Features of Preeclampsia
Hypertension	Blood pressure (BP) reading ≥140/90 mm Hg × 2, at least 4 hours apart after 20 weeks of gestation in a previously normotensive woman	BP reading ≥160/110 mm Hg × 2, at least 4 hours apart while the client is on bed rest (unless antihypertensive therapy has been initiated)
Proteinuria	Proteinuria of ≥300 mg in a 24-hr specimen Protein/creatinine ratio ≥0.3 (with each measured as mg/dL) ≥1+ on dipstick (used only if quantitative methods are not available)	Massive proteinuria (>5 g in a 24-hr specimen) is no longer used as a diagnostic criterion
Thrombocytopenia	Platelet count <100,000/μL	Platelet count <100,000/μL

Impaired liver function	Elevated blood levels of liver transaminases to twice the normal concentration	Abnormally elevated blood concentrations of liver enzymes to twice the normal concentration; severe persistent epigastric or right upper quadrant pain unresponsive to medication and not accounted for by alternative diagnoses, or both
Renal insufficiency	New development of serum creatinine >1.1 mg/dL or a doubling of the serum creatinine concentration in the absence of other renal disease	Progressive renal insufficiency (serum creatinine concentration >1.1 mg/dL or a doubling of the serum creatinine concentration in the absence of other renal disease
Pulmonary edema		Present
Cerebral or visual disturbances		New onset

Modified from American College of Obstetricians and Gynecologists (ACOG). (2013). Executive summary: Hypertension in pregnancy. *Obstetrics and Gynecology, 122* (5), 1122-1131.

Gestational Diabetes Mellitus Definition and Risk Factors

GDM is a carbohydrate intolerance of varying severity that develops during pregnancy and usually goes away after the birth of the baby.

Risk Factors

• Maternal age >30

• Obesity (>20% over ideal weight)

• Family history of NIDDM

• GDM in previous pregnancy

• Obstetrical history of large newborns (>9 lbs), stillbirths, miscarriages, hydramnios, or congenital anomalies

Gestational Diabetes Screen[42]

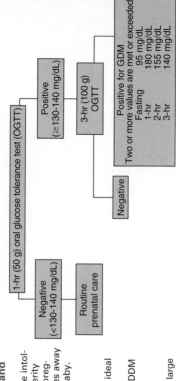

1-hr (50 g) oral glucose tolerance test (OGTT)

Negative (<130-140 mg/dL) → Routine prenatal care

Positive (≥130-140 mg/dL) → **3-hr (100 g) OGTT**

Negative

Positive for GDM
Two or more values are met or exceeded:

Fasting	95 mg/dL
1-hr	180 mg/dL
2-hr	155 mg/dL
3-hr	140 mg/dL

PEDIATRICS

Pediatrics

(Continued)

Drugs
  Emergency Drug Calculations
    for Children, *160*
Health Promotion
  Recommended Childhood and Adolescent
    Immunization Schedule—United States,
    2015, *161*
  Diet and Fitness, *162*

SEE ALSO

PROCEDURES

See for general Procedure information

LABS

See for pediatric Laboratory values

OBSTETRICS

Newborn
  APGAR Scoring System, *125*
  Vital Signs, *125*
  Initial Physical Assessment by Body
    System, *126*

Pediatrics

Airway and Gastric Equipment[59]

	Weight	Airway Oral/French (Nasal)	Endotracheal Tube Size	Laryngoscope Blade	French Catheter	Nasogastric Tube	Chest Tube
Newborn	2-3 kg/4.4-6.6 lb	00-2/10	2 5 uncuffed	0-1 straight	6	5-8	10-14
1-6 mo	4-7 kg/8.8-15.4 lb	00-2/10	3-3.5 uncuffed	1 straight	8	5-8	14-20
8 mo-1 yr	8-10 kg/17.6-22 lb	00-2/10	3.5-4.0 uncuffed	1 straight	8-10	8-10	14-24
2 yr	12 kg/26.4 lb	2-3/10-20	4.5 uncuffed	2 straight/curved	10	10	16-28
3-4 yr	14-16 kg/30.8-35.2 lb	2-3/10-20	4.5-5.0 uncuffed	2 straight/curved	10	10-12	16-30
5-7 yr	18-22 kg/39.6-48.4 lb	2-4/12-22	5-5.5 cuffed	2 straight/curved	10	12-14	16-32
7-10 yr	24-30 kg/52.8-66 lb	3-4/20-24	4.5-6.0 cuffed	2-3 straight/curved	10	14-18	28-38
10-12 yr	32-34 kg/70.4-74.8 lb	4-5/24-36	6.5 cuffed	4-5 straight/curved	10-16	18	38-42

Suctioning[51]

Note: Refer to procedures tab page 17 for basic procedure. The following apply to infants and children:

- Small-diameter suction catheter should be one-half the size of the child's tracheostomy tube.
- Use catheter with 3 holes
- Vacuum pressure should range from 60-100 mm Hg for infants and children and 40-60 mm Hg for premature infants.
- Distance suctioned should not be greater than the following:
  nasopharyngeal-
    older child 3 to 5 inches
    young child/infant 1.5 to 3 inches
  nasotracheal-
    older child 6 to 8 inches
    young child/infant 3 to 5 inches
  artificial airway- no greater than 0.25 to 0.5 inch beyond the tip of the artificial airway
- Suctioning should be limited to 5 sec for infants and 10 seconds for children

Intravenous Access[32]

- Pediatric veins are very fragile. Avoid sites that are easily moved or bumped.
- When possible, choose a site that does not interfere with activity, eating, or playing.
- When possible, avoid the child's dominant hand and avoid placement over a joint such as the antecubital fossa.
- If child is ambulatory, avoid foot/ankle.
- When starting an IV line, examine distal locations and then move proximal.
- A scalp or wrist vein may be used if a larger vein is not accessible.
- Most IV infusions require a 22- to 24-gauge catheter.

IM Injection Sites

If possible, administer **EMLA cream** or a topical vapocoolant spray to the injection site prior to the injection to decrease discomfort and pain.

Injection Sites[32]		
Age	**Preferred Muscle Group**	**Needle Length**
Infant <4 mo	Vastus lateralis	$5/8$ in
Infant 4 mo	Vastus lateralis	$5/8$ in
Toddler	Ventrogluteal or dorsogluteal >3 yr and walking 1 yr	1 in
Older child	Ventrogluteal	1-1.5 in

Vastus Lateralis Intramuscular Injection Site—Lateral Thigh[29]

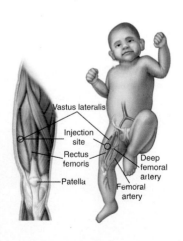

Labels: Vastus lateralis, Injection site, Rectus femoris, Patella, Deep femoral artery, Femoral artery

Preferred Sites for Intravenous Access in Infants[32]

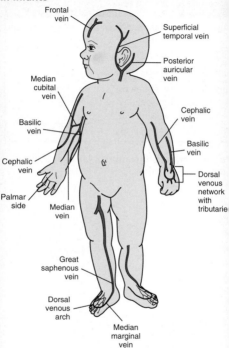

Frontal vein

Superficial temporal vein

Posterior auricular vein

Median cubital vein

Basilic vein

Cephalic vein

Cephalic vein

Basilic vein

Palmar side

Dorsal venous network with tributarie

Median vein

Great saphenous vein

Dorsal venous arch

Median marginal vein

Oxygen Administration[32]

System	Advantages	Disadvantages
Oxygen mask	• Various sizes available • Delivers higher level of O_2 than cannula • Provides predictable concentration for either nose- or mouth-breathing child	• Skin irritation/moisture on face • Fear of suffocation • Possibility of aspiration of vomitus • Difficulty controlling O_2 concentration
Nasal cannula	• Provides low-moderate oxygen concentration • Child can eat or talk while getting oxygen	• Must have patent nasal passages • Difficulty controlling O_2 level if mouth breather • Inability to provide mist
Oxygen tent	• Achieves lower O_2 concentration • Child receives increased inspired O_2 concentration even while eating	• Need tight fit around bed to prevent leaks • Cool and wet tent environment • Tent O_2 levels drop when tent entered
Oxygen hood, face tent	• Achieves high O_2 concentration • Easy access to chest for auscultation	• High humidity environment • Need to remove for feeding and care

VITAL SIGNS/PAIN[31]

Pediatric Vital Signs

Age	Weight (kg)	Heart Rate (average/min)	Respiratory Rate (average/min)	BP (sys) (mm Hg)
Premature	1	100-180	<40	42 ± 10
Newborn	2-3	100-180	<40	60 ± 10
1 mo	4	80-180	24-35	80 ± 16
6 mo	7	70-150	24-35	89 ± 29
1 yr	10	70-150	20-30	96 ± 30
2-3 yr	12-14	70-120	20-30	99 ± 25
4-5 yr	16-18	70-110	20-30	99 ± 20
6-8 yr	20-26	60-110	12-25	105 ± 13
10-12 yr	32-42	55-90	12-20	112 ± 19
>14 yr	>50	55-90	12-18	120 ± 20

PEDIATRIC PAIN ASSESSMENT

Wong-Baker FACES Pain Rating Scale

Brief word instructions: Point to each face using the words to describe the pain intensity. Ask the child to choose face that best describes his or her pain and record the appropriate number.

(From Hockenberry MJ: Wong's nursing care of infants and children, ed 10, St Louis, 2015, Mosby. Reprinted by permission.)

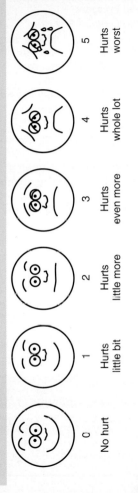

0	1	2	3	4	5
No hurt	Hurts little bit	Hurts little more	Hurts even more	Hurts whole lot	Hurts worst

Quick Formula for Determining Expected Blood Pressure

Systolic Blood Pressure

1-7 years:	age in years + 90
8-18 years:	$2 \times$ age in years + 83

Diastolic Blood Pressure

1-5 years:	56
6-18 years:	age in years + 52

Neonatal Pain Response

Physiologic

Vital signs: ↑ HR; ↑ BP; rapid, shallow respirations

Oxygenation: ↓ O_2 saturation

Skin: pallor or flushing; diaphoresis; palm sweating

Other: ↑ muscle tone; dilated pupils; ↓ vagal nerve tone

Behavioral

Vocalization: crying, whimpering, groaning

Facial expressions: grimaces, brows furrowed, chin quivering, eyes closed tightly mouth open

Body movement and posturing: limb withdrawal, thrashing, rigidity, flaccidity, fist clenching

Changes in: sleep, appetite, activity, affect

BLOOD GASES

Normal Values for Arterial Blood Gases[50]			
Parameter	**Neonate**	**2 mo-2 yr**	**>2 yr**
pH	7.32-7.49	7.34-7.46	7.35-7.45
Pco_2	26-41 mm Hg	26-41 mm Hg	35-45 mm Hg
HCO_3	16-24 mEq/L	21-28 mEq/L	21-28 mEq/L
Po_2	60-70 mm Hg	80-100 mm Hg	80-100 mm Hg

CIAMPEDS History[25]

	Format	Questions
C	Chief complaint	What brought the child to seek care? Current history of problem
I	Immunizations	Evaluation of child's exposure to communicable diseases Immunization history
A	Allergies	Evaluation of allergies to food, drugs, environment Describe type of reaction
M	Medications	Current medications Last dose: amount and time
P	Past medical history	Review of child's health status: prior illnesses, injuries, birth history and health since birth, hospitalization, surgery
E	Events surrounding the illness or injury	Evaluation of onset of illness or circumstances of injury
D	Diet	Assess diet history, fluid intake, urine and stool output; determine time and quantity of last intake and output
S	Symptoms associated with the illness or injury	Conduct symptom analysis

Growth and Development[24,25,32]

Age	Physical	Developmental Landmark
1 mo	Weight gain 5-7 oz weekly Height gain 1 in/mo Head circumference ↑ by 2 cm/3 mo Primitive reflexes present and strong Nose breathing	Lifts head while prone Regards other's face
2 mo	Posterior fontanel closes Crawling reflex disappears	Grasps rattle Coos/reciprocal vocalization Follows object 180 degrees Smiles responsively
4 mo	Primitive reflexes disappear: Moro, tonic neck, rooting Head circumference increases 1 cm Drooling begins	Holds head and neck up to make 90 degree angle Rolls prone to supine Hands midline Laughs/squeals Follows objects past midline

6 mo	Weight gain 3-5 oz/wk for next 6 mo Height gain 1/2 in monthly for next 6 mo Tooth eruption—2 lower incisors Chewing and biting occurs	No head lag if baby is pulled to sitting position Rolls from back to abdomen or vice versa Sits with a little support (one hand) Bears weight Reaches for object on table, raking pattern Turns toward sounds Babbles vowels Smiles spontaneously
9 mo	Visual acuity nears adult level Tooth eruption—upper lateral incisors Bowel and bladder function in regular pattern	Sits alone Crawls Pulls to standing position Stands holding on to solid object Has pincer grasp Tries to get toy just out of reach Transfers block from hand to hand Says "Da-da," "Ma-ma" Initial anxiety toward strangers Plays "peek-a-boo"

continued

Growth and Development (continued)

Age	Physical	Developmental Landmark
12 mo	Birth weight triples Birth length increases by 50% Has total of 6-8 deciduous teeth Anterior fontanel almost closed Head/chest circumference: 46 cm (18.1 in)	Stands alone 2-3 sec if outside support removed Walks around holding onto furniture Bangs 2 blocks together if held 1 in each hand Imitates vocalizing heard in preceding min Has 2-word vocabulary Waves bye-bye
15 mo	Steady growth in height and weight Head circumference: 48.3 cm (19 in) Weight: 10.9 kg (24 lb) Height: 31 in	Walks well Stoops to recover toys on floor Tries to feed self Uses "Da-da" and "Ma-ma" correctly Has 4- to 6-word vocabulary Indicates wants by pulling, pointing, or appropriate verbalization (not crying) Plays "pat-a-cake"

18 mo	Anterior fontanel closes Physiologically able to control sphincters	Walks up stairs with 1 hand held Puts 1 block on another without it falling off Rolls or tosses ball back to examiner Drinks from cup without spilling much; uses spoon Assists in removing clothing Has 6- to 10-word vocabulary Knows 1 body part Mimics household chores
2 yr	Head circumference: 48.3-50.8 cm (19.5-20 in) Chest circumference exceeds head circumference Usual weight gain 1.8-2.7 kg (4-6 lb) Weight: 11-12 kg (24.2-26.4 lb) Usual gain in height 4-5 in Primary dentition of 16 teeth	Goes up and down stairs holding a rail Kicks ball in front of self without support Balances 4 blocks on top of each other Dumps small object out of bottle after demonstration Scribbles spontaneously Combines 2 words Has 50-word vocabulary Points correctly to 5 parts of body Does simple tasks in house

continued

Growth and Development (continued)

Age	Physical	Developmental Landmark
2½ yr	Birth weight quadrupled Primary dentition of 20 teeth Some daytime bowel/bladder control	Throws overhand with demonstration Combines 2 words meaningfully Names correctly one picture in book (e.g., cat)
3 yr	Weight gain 1.8-2.7 kg (4-6 lb) Weight: 12-14 kg (26.4-30.8 lb) Average height growth 2.5-3 in/yr Average height: 37.25 in May have achieved nighttime control of bladder and bowel	Alternates feet ascending stairs Jumps in place; pedals tricycle Dumps small articles from bottle s̄ demonstration Copies circle Uses sentences intelligible to strangers Puts on clothing Washes and dries hands Knows name, sex, and age

4 yr	Weight: 16-17 kg (35.2-37.4 lb) Average height: 40.5 in Birth length is doubled	Alternates feet descending stairs Balances on 1 foot for 5 sec Builds bridge of 3 blocks after demonstration Copies circle and cross Identifies longer of 2 lines Cuts/pastes Dresses with supervision Plays with other children so they interact Knows first and last names
5 yr	Weight: 17-18.7 kg (37.4-41.2 lb) Average height: 43.25 in Eruption of permanent dentition may begin	Hops 2 or more times Imitates forward heel-to-toe walk Catches ball thrown 3 feet Draws 3-part person Dresses without supervision

continued

Age	Physical	Developmental Landmark
6 yr	Weight and height gain slows Weight: 19-24 kg (41.8-53 lb) Height: 42-48 in Central mandibular incisors erupt Gradual increase in dexterity	Performs backward heel-toe walk Copies a square; draws 6-part person Ties shoelaces Recognizes letters; writes name Defines 6 single words Names materials of which things are made
7 yr	Begins to grow 2 in/yr Weight: 24-30 kg (53-66 lb) Height: 44-51 in Maxillary central incisors and lateral mandibular incisors erupt More cautious in new activities	Copies a diamond Repeats 3 numbers backward Develops concept of time Likes to help, have a chore Is less resistant and stubborn Takes part in group play; prefers own gender

8-9 yr	Continues to grow 2 in/yr Weight: 26-39.5 kg (57.2-87 lb) Height: 46-56 in Lateral incisors/mandibular cuspids erupt	Counts backward from 20 to 1 Repeats days of weeks and months in order Enjoys reading more Helps with household tasks; runs errands Easy to get along with; more sociable Likes to compete and play games Plays mostly with same gender, begins to mix Likes school Sometimes critical of self
10-12 yr	Boys: slow growth in height; rapid weight gain Girls: pubescent changes may begin to appear Weight: 30-58.1 kg (66-128 lb) Height: 50-64 in Remainder of teeth erupt	Writes brief stories Reads for practical information Completes simple projects Successful in looking after own needs Loves friends Enjoys conversation Likes parents and wants to please them

Infant Reflexes[13]

Reflex	Description	Appearance	Disappearance
Babinski	Toes fan upward when sole of foot is stroked	Birth	9 mo
Galant	Arching of trunk toward stimulated side when infant is stroked along spine	Birth	Neonatal period
Moro (startle)	Sudden outward extension of arms with midline return when startled by loud noise or rapid change in position	Birth	4 mo
Palmar (grasp)	Grasping of object with fingers when palm is touched	Birth	4 mo
Parachute	Extension of arms and legs in protective manner when held in a horizontal prone and moving-downward position	8 mo	Indefinite
Plantar	Inward flexion of toes when balls of feet are stroked/touched	Birth	12 mo
Righting	Attempting to maintain head in upright position	Birth	24 mo
Rooting	Turning head toward stimulated side of cheek	Birth	6 mo
Sucking	Initiation of sucking when object is placed in mouth	Birth	Indefinite
Swimming	Mimicking swimming movement when held horizontally in water	Birth	4 mo
Walking	Making stepping movements when held upright with feet touching a surface	First weeks; reappears at 4-5 mo	12 mo

Degree of Dehydration[3,12]			
Signs and Symptoms	Mild (<5% loss)	Moderate (10% loss)	Severe (15% loss)
Mucous membranes	Somewhat dry	Dry	Dry, cracked
Skin turgor	Normal	Decreased (poor)	Very poor
Anterior fontanel	Normal	Sunken	Sunken
Eyes (appearance of)	Normal	Sunken	Sunken
Heart rate	Normal	Increased	Increased
Respiratory rate	Normal	Increased	Increased
Blood pressure	Normal	Minimally decreased	Decreased
Skin	Pale, warm	Very pale to cool, mottled	Mottled to cyanotic, cool
Capillary refill	Normal	Minimally delayed	Delayed
Mental status	Alert	Irritable	Lethargic

Breath Sound Abnormalities[26]

Breath Sound	Significance
Stridor, inspiratory crowing sound	Upper airway obstruction; high-pitched in croup and foreign body aspiration, low-pitched and muffled in epiglottitis
Wheezing, usually inspiratory but may be expiratory	Lower airway obstruction; bilateral wheezing suggests asthma or bronchiolitis; unilateral wheezing suggests foreign body aspiration
Decreased or unequal breath sounds	Airway obstruction, pneumothorax, pleural effusion, pneumonia
Grunting	Early closure of the glottis during exhalation with active chest wall contraction; increases expiratory airway pressure, preventing airway collapse; creates PEEP; seen in diseases with diminished lung compliance such as pulmonary edema; also occurs as a result of pain

Clinical Signs of Respiratory Failure[32]

Cardinal Signs

- Restlessness
- Tachypnea
- Tachycardia
- Diaphoresis

Early but Less Obvious Signs

- Mood changes—euphoria or depression
- Headache
- Altered depth and pattern of respirations
- Hypertension
- Exertional dyspnea
- Anorexia
- Increased cardiac and renal output
- Central nervous symptoms (eg: impaired judgement, confusion, restlessness, irritability)
- Nasal flaring, chest wall retractions,
- Expiratory grunting,
- Wheezing or prolonged expiration

Signs of More Severe Hypoxia

- Hypotension
- Depressed respirations, dyspnea
- Dimness of vision
- Bradycardia, arrythmias
- Somnolence
- Cyanosis
- Stupor, coma

Physical Abuse[32]

Physical Findings	Suggestive Behaviors
• Bruises and welts, in different stages of healing	• Wariness of physical contact with adults
• Burns, especially on feet, palms of hands, back and buttocks; patterns descriptive of object used (eg: round cigarette burns, rope burns on wrists/ankles)	• Apparent fear of parent or of going home
	• Lying very still while surveying environment
	• Inappropriate reaction to injury such as failure to cry from pain
• Fractures/dislocations—skull, nose, facial; spiral fracture/dislocation; old fractures in various healing stages	• Lack of reactions to frightening events
	• Superficial relationships
	• Indiscriminate displays of affection
• Lacerations/abrasions on back of arms, torso, face, or external genitalia; bites or pulling out of hair	• Anxiety when hearing other children cry
• Unexplained poisonings	• Withdrawal or acting out behavior
• Unexplained sudden illness (eg: hypoglycemia from insulin dosing)	

Physical Neglect[32]

Physical Findings	Suggestive Behaviors
• Growth Failure	• Dull and inactive, passive or sleepy
• Malnutrition, lack of subcutaneous fat	• Self-stimulation, (eg: finger sucking, rocking)
• Poor personal hygiene	• Begging/stealing food
• Unclean and/or inappropriate dress	• Absenteeism from school
• Poor health care	• Substance abuse
• Frequent illnesses or injury	• Vandalism/shoplifting

Emotional Abuse/Neglect[32]

Physical Findings	Suggestive Behaviors
• Growth failure • Eating/feeding disorders • Enuresis • Sleep disorders	• Self-stimulatory behaviors (eg: finger sucking, rocking, biting) • No social smile, stranger anxiety in infants • Unusual fearfulness • Antisocial behavior/behavior extremes • Lag in emotional or intellectual development • Suicide attempts

Sexual Abuse[32]

Physical Findings	Suggestive Behaviors
• Bruises, bleeding, lacerations or irritation to external genitalia, anus, mouth, or throat • Torn, stained, bloody underclothing • Pain on urination or pain, swelling, and itching of genital area • Penile discharge • Sexually transmitted infection, nonspecific vaginitis • Difficulty walking or sitting • Unusual odor in genital area • Recurrent urinary tract infection • Presence of semen • Pregnancy in young adolescent	• Sudden emergence of sexually related problems, sexual play, excessive masturbation, seductive behavior • Withdrawn behavior, excessive daydreaming • Preoccupation with fantasies • Poor relationship with peers • Sudden changes (eg: anxiety, weight loss/gain, clinging behavior) • Regressive behaviors-bedwetting, thumb sucking • Running away from home • Substance abuse • Profound and rapid personality changes • Suicide attempts or ideation

BLS Guidelines for Cardiopulmonary Arrest — Infant/Child[1,4]

CPR	1 to 12 years	Under 1 year
Assess unresponsiveness	Attempt to arouse • If responsive CPR not needed • If unresponsive and no breathing or gasping detected, have someone activate ERS and get defibrillator*	
Check pulse	Palpate Carotid artery • If pulse present, begin breathing • If no pulse, start compressions	Palpate Brachial or femoral artery • If pulse present, begin breathing • If no pulse, start compressions
Provide compressions	• Just below nipple line • Use heel of hand • Depth 1.5 to 2 inches	• Just below nipple line • Use 2 fingers • 1 to 1.5 inches

Compression rate	• Compress at rate of 100/min • Push fast for 30 compressions then open the airway
Open airway/ Breathe	• Use head tilt/chin lift position. If trauma suspected, use a jaw thrust only • Give 2 breaths. Chest should rise and fall with each breath. Avoid overventilation (too many breaths or too much volume)
Compression: ventilation ratio	30:2 (deliver 30 compressions, then 2 breaths)
Assess cardiac rhythm	When defibrillator is available, assess for shockable rhythm • If rhythm is not shockable, continue CPR and reassess rhythm every 5 cycles • If rhythm is shockable, defibrillate
Defibrillate	• Use an AED with a pediatric attenuated pads • Deliver 1 shock, then resume CPR for 5 cycles, then reassess rhythm • Manual defibrillator is preferred. Or use AED equipped with a pediatric attenuated pads • Deliver 1 shock and resume CPR for 5 cycles, then reassess rhythm

*A lone rescuer should perform 5 cycles of CPR (about 30 compressions and 2 breaths for about 2 min) before leaving an infant or child victim to activate the emergency response system and obtain an AED.

BLS Guidelines for Relief of Foreign-Body Airway Obstruction (Choking)—Infant/Child[11]

Victim	8 years and older	1 to 8 years	Younger than 1 year
Responsive	Can child speak or cough? • If yes, do not interfere, observe for worsening obstruction • If no, perform up to 5 subdiaphragmatic abdominal thrusts	Can child speak or cough? • If yes, do not interfere, observe for worsening obstruction	Can infant cry or effectively breathe? • If yes, continue to observe • If no, give 5 back blows then 5 chest thrusts
	Repeat actions until obstruction is relieved or victim becomes unconscious		
Becomes unresponsive	Place victim on back Send someone to activate EMS		
	• Start CPR with 30 chest compressions (do not perform pulse check) • Open airway and remove foreign body if seen (do not perform a blind sweep) • Give 2 rescue breaths then 30 chest compressions		
	Continue 30:2 cycle of compressions and ventilations until object is expelled		
	After 2 minutes if no one has done so, activate EMS		

Pediatric Modification of Glasgow Coma Scale by Age of Patient[12]

	0-1 yr	Older than 1 yr	Older than 5 yr
Eye Opening	4 Spontaneously 3 To shout 2 To pain 1 No response	4 Spontaneously 3 To verbal command 2 To pain 1 No response	4 Spontaneously 3 To verbal command 2 To pain 1 No response
Best Motor Response	6 Normal spontaneous movements 5 Localizes pain 4 Flexion withdrawal 3 Flexion abnormal (decorticate) 2 Extension (decerebrate) 1 No response	6 Obeys 5 Localizes pain 4 Flexion withdrawal 3 Flexion abnormal (decorticate) 2 Extension (decerebrate) 1 No response	6 Obeys 5 Localizes pain 4 Flexion withdrawal 3 Flexion abnormal 2 Extension 1 No response

	0-2 yr	2-5 yr	Older than 5 yr
Best Verbal Response	5 Cries appropriately, smiles, coos 4 Cries 3 Inappropriate crying/screaming 2 Grunts 1 No response	5 Appropriate words and phrases 4 Inappropriate words 3 Cries/screams 2 Grunts 1 No response	5 Oriented and converses 4 Disoriented and converses 3 Inappropriate words 2 Incomprehensible sounds 1 No response

Emergency Drug Calculations for Children

Drug (concentration)	Dose in mg
Epinephrine 1:10,000 (0.1 mg/mL)	0.01 mg/kg = ___ mg
Epinephrine 1:1000 (1.0 mg/mL)	0.1 mg/kg = ___ mg
Atropine (0.1 mg/mL)	0.02 mg/kg = ___ mg (maximum dose = 0.5 mg, minimum dose = 0.1 mg)
CaCl$_2$ 10% (100 mg/mL)	20 mg/kg = ___ mg
Adenosine (3 mg/mL)	0.1 mg/kg = ___ mg
Dextrose 25% (25 g/100 mL) (dilute D$_{50}$ 1:1 with sterile H$_2$0)	0.5 g/kg = ___ gm (up to 1 g/kg)
Na bicarb (1 mEq/mL) (dilute 1:1 with saline)	1 mEq/kg = ___ mEq
Naloxone (1 mg/mL)	0.1 mg/kg = ___ mg
Lorazepam (4 mg/mL)	0.1 mg/kg = ___ mg
Diazepam (5 mg/mL)	0.2 mg/kg = ___ mg (slow IV push, undiluted up to 0.4 mg/kg/dose)

Vaccine ▼ Age ►	Birth	1 mo	2 mo	4 mo	6 mo	12 mo	15 mo	18 mo	19-23 mo	2-3 yrs	4-6 yrs	7-10 yrs	11-12 yrs	13-18 yrs
Hepatitis B	HepB	HepB			Hep3							HepB series		
Rotavirus			RV	RV	RV									
Diphtheria, Tetanus, Pertussis			DTaP	DTaP	DTaP		DTaP				DTaP		Tdap	Tdap
Haemophilus influenzae type b			Hib	Hib	Hib	Hib								
Pneumococcal			PCV	PCV	PCV	PCV				PPSV			Pneumococcal	
Inactivated Poliovirus			IPV	IPV		IPV					IPV		IPV series	
Influenza						Influenza (Yearly)								
Measles, Mumps, Rubella						MMR					MMR		MMR series	
Varicella						Varicella					Varicella		Varicella series	
Hepatitis A						HepA (2 doses)				HepA Series				
Meningococcal										MCV4	MCV4		MCV4	MCV4
Papillomavirus													HPV ♀ (3 doses)	HPV series

Consult www.cdc.gov and the Manufacturer's package for full details.

■ Range of recommended ages ■ Range for certain high-risk groups ■ Catch-up immunization

Diet and Fitness

Nutrition—Maintain calorie balance				
Fruits =Focus on fruits—1 to 2 cups a day (↑ with age)	**Vegetables** Vary your veggies— 1-3 cups a day (↑ with age)	**Grains** Make half your grains whole 5-8 oz. a day (↑ with age)	**Protein** Go lean with protein— 4-6 oz. a day (↑ with age)	**Dairy** Get your calcium rich foods 2.5-3 cups a day

Oils provide essential nutrients—use oil from fish, nuts and liquid oils. Decrease saturated fats.

Physical Activity—at least 60 minutes a day	
Aerobic: rhythmic movement of large muscles (eg: hop, run, skip, dance, bike, swim) moderate to vigorous-intensity needed daily.	**Muscle Strengthening:** make muscles work hard (eg: climb, play tug of war, use resistance bands, lift heavy objects) needed at least 3 days a week
	Bone Strengthening: place force on large bones (eg: run, hop, jump rope, play basketball, play tennis) needed at least 3 days a week

Modified from _Incorporate to go_ USDA _ds..mygmlate.gov_

GERIATRICS

SEE ALSO

PROCEDURES

ee for general Procedures information

VITAL SIGNS/ASSESSMENT

ee for general Vital Signs/Assessment
information

Geriatrics

ELDER RESOURCES

Organizations

Administration on Aging
www.aoa.gov
Alzheimer's Association
www.alz.org
American Association of Retired Persons
www.aarp.org
American Geriatrics Society
www.americangeriatrics.org
American Society on Aging
www.asaging.org
Clearinghouse of Abuse and Neglect of the Elderly
www.elderabusecenter.org/clearing
Senior Initiative in Consumer Law
www.consumerlaw.org
Gerontological Society of America
www.geron.org
National Council on Aging
www.ncoa.org
National Gerontological Nursing Association
www.ngna.org
National Institute on Aging
www.nia.nih.gov

Journals/Periodicals

Generations
www.asaging.org/generations-journal
-american-society-aging
Geriatric Nursing
www.journals.elsevierhealth.com
Journal of Gerontological Nursing
www.slackinc.com/jgn.htm

Educational Resources

ElderWeb
www.elderweb.com
GeroNet Health & Aging Services
www.geronet.ucla.edu

Vital Signs in Older Adults

VITAL SIGN	NORMAL VALUES	ASSESSMENT/PROCEDURE CONSIDERATIONS
Temperature	• Average oral temp in those >75 yr is 97.2° F (36° C).	• Electronic thermometers are preferred to ↓ procedure time. • Oral route most common; missing teeth, weak oral muscles may interfere with holding probe. • Earwax may interfere with tympanic route. • Use rectal route with caution; tissue is fragile.
Pulse	• Normal range is 50-90. • Normal pulse rate is lower at rest. • Once ↑, rate takes longer to retu'n to resting rate.	• Radial artery is most common site. • Use gentle palpation to prevent occlusion of the vessel. • If pulse is difficult to feel, use Doppler stethoscope. • Apical pulse should be taken regularly.
Respirations	• Lower normal range is 12. • ↓ in resting rate may be a sign of impending infection. • ↑ rates common with anxiety, activity, illness.	• Chest wall movement and depth of respirations are ↓; watch rise and fall of abdomen to assist in count. • Count for a full minute.
Blood pressure	• Systolic pressure tends to ↑ with age. • Upper range of normal is 150. • BP varies widely.	• Use same position for each reading; susceptible to posture-related changes. • Select appropriate cuff size; upper arm mass is reduced. • Avoid pumping cuff to excessively high pressures. • Assess skin under cuff for bruising.

Assessment of Age-Related Changes in Key Body Systems[35,66]

SYSTEM	AGE-RELATED CHANGES	ASSESSMENT
Eyes	↓ tearing, ↑ sensitivity to light, ↓ corneal sensitivity, ↓ depth perception, ↓ peripheral vision; presbyopia, glaucoma, cataracts	Any difficulty seeing, reading, driving, seeing at night, stepping up or down? Eyes dry/burning, light sensitivity? ✓ for low vision aids
Ears	Hearing loss (conductive and sensorineural), ↑ earwax, ↑ time to process/respond to sound	Any difficulty hearing? Dizziness? Trouble with balance? ✓ for hearing aid
Skin	Skin is drier, thinner, fragile; senile and seborrheic keratoses, skin tags; nails thicker, brittle	Delay in wound healing? Itching/dry skin? Nails trimmed? ✓ skin for bruises, reddened areas, hydration
Mouth	Yellowing teeth, receding gums, loss of taste buds; dentures	Any change in ability to chew? Taste of food? Appetite? Ability to swallow? ✓ for dentures, feeding tube
Bladder/bowels	↓ GI peristalsis; ↓ tone in bladder muscles	Trouble urinating? Incontinence? Leaking? Nocturia? Constipation?
Musculoskeletal	Loss of bone density and muscle mass; worn cartilage in joints; ↓ mobility	Trouble walking, climbing stairs, sitting, or getting up? Joints stiff, painful? ✓ for mobility aids
Neurologic	↓ reaction time; dizziness/loss of balance with quick movement	Trouble with memory? Confusion? Dizziness? Tremor? LOC? ✓ orientation

Hendrich II Fall Risk Model[5]

K FACTOR	RISK POINTS	SCORE
nfusion/Disorientation/Impulsivity	4	
nptomatic Depression	2	
ered Elimination	1	
ziness/Vertigo	1	
nder (Male)	1	
y Administered Antiepileptics (anticonvulsants): rbamazepine, Divalproex Sodium, Ethotoin, Ethosuximide, bamate, Fosphenytoin, Gabapentin, Lamotrigine, ohenytoin, Methsuximide, Phenobarbital, Phenytoin, nidone, Topiramate, Trimethadi-one, Valproic Acid)[1]	2	
y Administered Benzodiazepines:[2] orazolam, Chloridiazepoxide, Clonazepam, Clorazepate otassium, Diazepam, Flurazepam, Halazepam[3], azepam, Midazolam, Oxazepam, Temazepam, Triazolam)	1	
t-Up-and-Go Test: "Rising from a Chair" nable to assess, monitor for change in activity level, assess other risk factors, ument both on patient chart with date and time.		
lity to rise in single movement - No loss of ance with steps	0	
shes up, successful in one attempt	1	
ltiple attempts but successful	3	
able to rise without assistance during test nable to assess, document this on the patient chart n the date and time.	4	
score of 5 or greater = High Risk)	**TOTAL SCORE**	

-going Medication Review Updates:

evetiracetam (Keppra) was not assessed during the original research nducted to create the Hendrich Fall Risk Model. As an antiepileptic, vetiracetam does have a side effect of somnolence and dizziness hich contributes to its fall risk and should be scored (effective June 010).

he study did not include the effect of benzodiazepine-like drugs since ey were not on the market at the time. However, due to their similarity drug structure, mechanism of action and drug effects, they should so e scored (effective January 2010).

alazepam was included in the study but is no longer available in the nited States (effective June 2010).

Six-Item Cognitive Impairment Test

Item	Maximum Error	Score	Weight	Final Item Score
1. What year is it now?	1		4	
2. What month is it now?	1		3	
Memory phrase: Repeat this phrase after me: "John Brown, 42 Market Street, Chicago"				
3. About what time is it now? (within an hour)	1		3	
4. Count backwards 20 to 1	2		2	
5. Say the months in reverse order	2		2	
6. Repeat the memory phrase	5		2	

Mental Status Assessment[14]

Assign 0 for a correct score, and 1 for each incorrect score up to the maximum number of errors permitted. Multiply the item score by the item weight to obtain the final item score. The maximum total score possible is 28. A score of 10 or higher is significant and should be referred.

168

Functional Assessment

ACTIVITY TO OBSERVE	INDICATORS OF WEAKENED MUSCLE GROUPS
Rising from lying to sitting position	Rolling to one side and pushing with arms to raise to elbows; grabbing side rail or table to pull to sitting position
Rising from chair to standing	Pushing with arms to supplement weak leg muscles; upper torso thrusts forward before body rises
Walking	Lifting leg farther off floor with each step; shortened swing phase; foot may fall or slide forward; arms held out for balance or move in rowing motion
Climbing steps	Holding handrail for balance; pulling body up and forward with arms; uses stronger leg
Descending steps	Lowering weakened leg first; often descends sideways holding rail with both hands; may watch feet
Tying shoes	Using footstool to decrease spinal flexion

continued

Functional Assessment (continued)

Picking up item from floor	Leaning on furniture for support; bending over at waist to avoid bending knees; using one hand on thigh to assist with lowering and raising torso
Putting on and pulling up trousers or stockings	Difficulty may indicate decreased shoulder and upper arm strength; these activities often performed in sitting position until clothing is pulled up
Putting on sweater	Putting sleeve on weaker arm or shoulder first; uses internal or external shoulder rotation to get remaining arm in sleeve
Zipping dress in back	Difficulty with this indicates weakened shoulder rotation
Combing hair	Difficulty indicates problems with grasp, wrist flexion, pronation and supination of forearm, and elbow rotation
Pushing chair away from table while seated	Standing and easing chair back with torso; difficulty indicates problems with upper arm, shoulder, lower arm strength, and wrist motion
Buttoning button or writing name	Difficulty indicates problem with manual dexterity and finger-thumb opposition

Independence in Activities of Daily Living (ADL) Scale[66]

ACTIVITIES	SCORE (0 TO 4)
Bathing	0 1 2 3 4
Hygiene (e.g., shave, comb hair, brush teeth)	0 1 2 3 4
Toileting	0 1 2 3 4
Continence	0 1 2 3 4
Dressing	0 1 2 3 4
Transferring	0 1 2 3 4
Ambulating	0 1 2 3 4
Feeding	0 1 2 3 4
Total Score (0-24)	

°y:
= Completely independent
= Requires devices or equipment
= Requires supervision, direction, or assistance
= Requires both devices and assistance
- Totally dependent
e higher the score, the more assistance needed.

Elder Abuse Assessment[67]

1. Has anyone close to you tried to hurt or harm you recently?
2. Do you feel uncomfortable with anyone in your family?
3. Does anyone tell you that you give them too much trouble?
4. Has anyone forced you to do things that you didn't want to do?
5. Has anyone taken things that belong to you without your okay?
6. Do you feel that nobody wants you around?
7. Does someone else make decisions about your life, such as how or where you should live?
8. Has anyone close to you called you names or put you down or made you feel bad recently?
   A "yes" to any question indicates a need for further assessment.

Modified Hwalek-Sengstock Elder Abuse Screening Test H-S/EAST).

Norton Scale for Assessing Risk of Pressure Ulcers[45]

Name	Date	Physical Condition		Mental Condition		Activity		Mobility		Incontinent		Total Score
		Good	4	Alert	4	Ambulant	4	Full	4	Not	4	
		Fair	3	Apathetic	3	Walk/help	3	Slightly Limited	3	Occasional	3	
		Poor	2	Confused	2	Chairbound	2	Very Limited	2	Usually/urine	2	
		Bad	1	Stupor	1	Bedridden	1	Immobile	1	Doubly	1	

The Norton Scale uses five criteria to assess patients' risk for pressure ulcers. Scores of 14 or less indicate susceptibility to ulcers; scores of <12 indicate very high risk.

172

Pressure Ulcer Stages

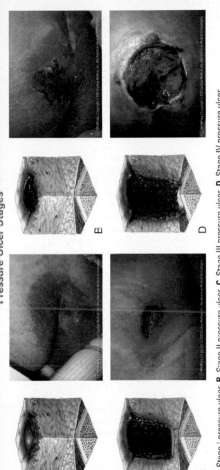

A, Stage I pressure ulcer. **B,** Stage II pressure ulcer. **C,** Stage III pressure ulcer. **D,** Stage IV pressure ulcer.

Use of Restraints[66]

When (all the following are necessary):
- Person is at serious risk for self-harm or a threat to others
- All other alternative methods have failed
- A physician order is in place
- Informed consent is signed by patient/guardian

What:
- Least restrictive device that allows greatest level of function while providing level of protection required

How:
- Inspect skin where restraint is to be placed
- Place patient in correct position
- Pad bony prominences
- Apply restraint according to manufacturer's instructions and agency policy
- Allow two fingers of space under restraint
- Be sure restraint does not interfere with other equipment (IV tubing, catheters, etc.)
- Attach restraint to chair/bed frame (not side rails)
- Secure with quick-release knots
- Place call bell within reach
- Check patient frequently
- Release restraints and inspect area beneath restraint at least every 2 hrs

Restraint Alternatives[54]

- Frequent orientation to surroundings
- Adequate supervision (e.g., use of sitters)
- Redirection and reorientation
- Reminiscence
- Visual and auditory stimuli for orientation (e.g., clocks, calendar, family pictures)
- Scheduled toileting routines
- Enhance ADLs
- Exercise, strength training
- Ambialarms, identabands
- Secure exits

Med Abuse Patterns in the Older Adult[54]

Polypharmacy: use of numerous simultaneous meds to treat chronic conditions. This increases the likelihood of drug interactions and adverse drug effects while decreasing drug effectiveness

Self-prescription: use of over-the-counter (OTC) meds, folk meds, herbal remedies, and prescription meds to treat common problems such as pain, constipation, insomnia, indigestion, cold symptoms

Medication misuse: taking doses at the wrong time, in the wrong amount, by the wrong route; taking the wrong meds; omitting doses of meds; using inappropriate procedures to administer meds

Medication noncompliance: deliberate misuse/nonuse of meds due to side effects, finances, med ineffectiveness

Tips for Administering Meds to Older Adults[54]

Space oral meds so that the patient takes no more than one or two at one time.

Have patient drink a little fluid before taking oral meds (to ease swallowing).

Encourage the patient to drink at least 5 or 6 ounces of fluid after taking meds (to ensure that the meds have left the esophagus and are in the stomach and to speed absorption of the meds).

Do not routinely give analgesics for pain q4h. Delayed absorption/distribution may cause an adverse cumulative effect.

If patient has difficulty swallowing large capsules or tablet, ask physician to substitute a liquid med if possible. Do not break or crush tablets; do not place tablets in food or juice as it may distort med action or cause choking.

Teach alternatives to meds, such as the following:

► Proper diet instead of vitamins
► Exercise instead of laxatives
► Bedtime snacks instead of hypnotics
► Decrease weight, salt, fat intake, stress; cease smoking; increase exercise to decrease BP.

Examples of Inappropriate Medications for Older Adults*[22]

GENERIC NAME	BRAND NAME
Avoid	
Barbiturates	Seconal, Nembutal
Belladonna alkaloids	Donnatal
Chlorpropamide	Diabinese
Dicyclomine	Bentyl
Flurazepam	Dalmane
Hyoscyamine	Levsin, Levsinex
Meprobamate	Equanil, Miltown
Meperidine	Demerol
Pentazocine	Talwin
Propantheline	Pro-Banthine
Trimethobenzamide	Tigan
Rarely appropriate	
Carisoprodol	Soma
Chlordiazepoxide	Librium, Librax
Chlorzoxazone	Paraflex
Cyclobenzaprine	Flexeril
Diazepam	Valium
Dipyridamole	Persantine
Metaxalone	Skelaxin
Methocarbamol	Robaxin
Nifedipine (short acting)	Procardia
Propranolol	Inderal
Sometimes indicated	
Amitriptyline	Elavil
Chlorpheniramine	Chlor-Trimeton
Cyproheptadine	Periactin
Diphenhydramine	Benadryl
Disopyramide	Norpace, Norpace CR
Doxepin	Sinequan
Hydroxyzine	Vistaril, Atarax
Methyldopa	Aldomet
Promethazine	Phenergan
Reserpine	Serpasil
Ticlopidine	Ticlid

*For a complete listing of inappropriate medications, 2015 updated Beers criteria list at http://onlinelibrary.wiley.com/doi/10.1111/jgs.13702/pdf.

HEALTH MAINTENANCE

TEN ACTIONS FOR A HEALTHIER YOU

. Eat a balanced diet.

. Stay active.

. Get adequate quantity/quality sleep every night.

. Manage your stress level and have fun.

. Do not smoke.

. Drink alcohol in moderation or not at all.

. Maintain your weight within a normal range.

. Nurture relationships with family and friends.

. Practice good physical and sexual hygiene.

. Seek regular health care.

Health
Maintenance

ACTIVITY/EXERCISE

Physical Activity Pyramid—Adult[16]

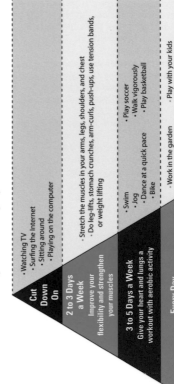

Cut Down On
- Watching TV
- Surfing the Internet
- Sitting around
- Playing on the computer

2 to 3 Days a Week
Improve your flexibility and strengthen your muscles
- Stretch the muscles in your arms, legs, shoulders, and chest
- Do leg-lifts, stomach crunches, arm-curls, push-ups, use tension bands, or weight lifting

3 to 5 Days a Week
Give your heart and lungs a workout with aerobic activity
- Swim
- Jog
- Dance at a quick pace
- Bike
- Play soccer
- Walk vigorously
- Play basketball

Every Day
Walk often and be physically active
- Work in the garden
- Rake leaves
- Play with your kids
- Walk to work

Levels of Physical Activity[62]

- Baseline activity—light-intensity activities of daily life (e.g., standing, walking slowly, lifting light objects)
- Moderate-intensity activity—physical activity that burns 3.5-7 kcal/min (e.g., brisk walking, jumping rope, dancing, yoga, bicycling, calisthenics)
- Vigorous-intensity activity—physical activity that burns greater than 7 kcal/min (e.g., running, climbing, cross-country skiing, high-impact aerobics)

Health Benefits of Activity[62]

Activity Level	Mod Intensity Activities Min/wk	Overall Health Benefit
Inactive	None beyond baseline activity	None
Low	Less than 150 min/wk hear	Some
Medium	150-300 min/wk	Substantial
High	More than 300 min/wk	Additional

Exercise Prescription[62]

- When initiating an exercise program, start slowly and build time and intensity each week until hitting recommended weekly time targets.
- Adults should accumulate at least 150 minutes or more of moderate-intensity activity per week.
- This amount of activity should expend a minimum of 750 to 1500 calories per week.
- The activity need not be continuous; benefits can be realized with short bouts of activity (a minimum of 10 minutes).

NUTRITION

Nutritional Self-Assessment Tool[24]

Check each statement that describes the way you usually eat.

1. I take the time to fully enjoy my food. I pay attention to hunger and fullness cues.
2. I know how to balance calories between my portions and my activity levels.
3. I avoid oversized portions.
4. Most days of the week, I make vegetables, fruits, whole grains, and no or low-fat dairy products the foundation for my meals and snacks.
5. I eat small servings of meat, poultry, and fish (no larger than the size of a deck of cards), or I do not eat meat and substitute other protein sources such as eggs, beans, legumes, or nuts/seeds.
6. I make fruits and vegetables half of my plate at most meals with a variety of types and colors.
7. I have switched to low-fat milk and dairy products or the equivalent substitutes (e.g., almond or soy milk).
8. I eat grains daily (such as bread, cereal, pasta, rice) and normally make half of them whole grains.
9. I use unsaturated liquid oils (e.g., olive, canola, safflower, or corn) rather than saturated or trans fats.
10. I substitute water or unsweetened beverages for sugary drinks (soda, energy drinks, and sports drinks).
11. I compare sodium levels in foods to choose lower-sodium versions (e.g., soup, bread, frozen meals, and canned products).
12. I do not drink alcohol, or I drink no more than 1 to 2 beers, 1 to 2 glasses of wine, or 1 to 2 mixed drinks daily.

Add up the number of statements checked:

Score: 9 to 12 Great job! Keep up the good work.
Score: 5 to 8 Okay. You make some good choices, but food habits need to be fine-tuned.

Score: 0 to 4 Improvement needed. Full dietary assessment and overhaul recommended.

Nutrition

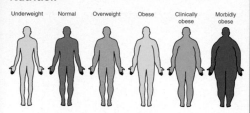

Underweight · Normal · Overweight · Obese · Clinically obese · Morbidly obese

Classification of Overweight and Obesity by BMI, Waist Circumference, and Associated Disease Risks[47]

	BMI (kg/m²)	Disease Risk* Relative to BMI and Waist Circumference	
		Waist less than or equal to 40 inches (men) 35 inches (women)	Waist greater than 40 inches (men) 35 inches (women)
Underweight	< 18.5	–	–
Normal	18.5–24.9	–	–
Overweight	25.0–29.9	Increased	High
Obesity	30.0–34.9	High	Very high
	35.0–39.9	Very high	Very high
Extreme obesity	40.0 +	Extremely high	Extremely high

* Disease risk for type 2 diabetes, hypertension, and CVD.
† Increased waist circumference also can be a marker for increased risk, even in persons of normal weight.

Calculation of BMI

$$BMI = \frac{Weight\ (lb) \times 705}{Height\ (inches)^2} \quad or \quad BMI = \frac{Weight\ (kg)}{Height\ (m)^2}$$

MyPlate Sample Foods

Grains Make half your grains whole	Vegetables Vary your veggies	Fruits Focus on fruits	Dairy Get your calcium-rich foods	Protein Go lean with protein
Increase whole grains (e.g., oatmeal, brown rice, whole wheat, popcorn). Reduce refined grains (e.g., white rice, white bread, cornmeal, pasta).	Eat more dark green veggies (e.g., spinach, broccoli, kale). Eat more red/orange veggies (e.g., carrots, sweet potatoes, tomatoes, red peppers).	Eat a variety of fruit. Chose fresh, frozen, canned, or dried fruit. Go easy on fruit juices.	Go low-fat or fat-free with dairy products (e.g., milk, yogurt, cheese). If you can't consume milk, select other calcium sources (e.g., lactose-free milk, rice milk, soy milk).	Choose lean meats, poultry, seafood. Bake, broil, or grill it. Try varied sources (beans, peas, nuts, seeds).

Amounts of foods needed depend on age, sex, and physical activity. Recommendations below are for an adult who gets less than 30 minutes of exercise daily. For more specific information, go to www.choosemyplate.gov

Grains	Vegetables	Fruits	Dairy	Protein
6 oz a day	2.5 cups a day	2 cups a day	3 cups a day	5.5 oz a day

Find your balance between food and physical activity

- Be sure to stay within your daily calorie needs.
- Be physically active for at least 30 minutes most days of the week.
- About 60 minutes a day of physical activity may be needed to prevent weight gain.
- For sustaining weight loss, at least 60 to 90 minutes a day of physical activity may be required.
- Children and teenagers should be physically active for 60 minutes every cay, or most days.

Know the limits on fats, sugars, and salt (sodium)

- Make fish, nuts, and vegetable oils your main sources of fat.
- Limit solid fats like butter, stick margarine, shortening, and lard, as well as foods that contain these.
- Check the Nutrition Facts label to keep saturated fats, trans fats, and sodium low.
- Choose food and beverages low in added sugars. Added sugars contribute calories with few, if any, nutrients.

MyPyramid.gov

182

Sleep Requirements[30]	
AGE	**SLEEP NEEDS**
Infants	12-15 hrs
Toddlers 1-2 yr	11-14 hrs
Preschool 3-5 yr	10-13 hrs
School age 6-13 yr	9-11 hrs
Teens 14-17 yr	8-10 hrs
Adults 18-64 yr	7-9 hrs
Older Adults >64 yr	7-8 hrs

Sleep Hygiene Strategies

- Establish a regular relaxing bedtime routine; avoid daytime naps.
- Associate your bed with sleep (e.g., don't read or watch TV in bed).
- Bedroom should be quiet, cool, and dark.
- Avoid large meals and stimulants (e.g., caffeine, nicotine, alcohol) before bedtime.
- Perform vigorous exercise in morning or afternoon. Relaxing exercise (e.g., yoga, stretching) can promote restful sleep

STRESS MANAGEMENT

Mini Relaxation Exercise (Mini)

- Start by recalling an image that brings a smile to your face.
- Inhale slowly through your nose and exhale through your mouth.
- Count to 4 as you inhale and back down to 1 as you exhale.
- Repeat 5-10 times.

Laughter Exercise

- Fake a smile.
- Giggle.
- Laugh, slowly increasing the volume.
- Build the laugh to a deep belly laugh.

General Health Screening Recommendations[63,64]

Tests	Screening Recommendations
Physical exam including height, weight	Every 5 yr (20-29); every 1-5 yr (30-64); annually (65 and ↑)
Blood pressure	If BP is < 120/80, every 2 yr. If slightly elevated (120-130/80-89), check annually
Cholesterol	If normal, every 5 yr (start at age 34 in males and age 45 in females)
Dental exam	Annually
Eye exam	If normal, every 2 yr after age of 40; add glaucoma checks after age 45.
Hearing exam	Baseline at 20; every 10 yr (30-49); every 3 yr (50-64); annually (65 and ↑)
Blood glucose/A1c test	Baseline at 45; then every 3 yr
Bone density scan (DEXA scan)	Women: all postmenopausal women with a fracture; all women over age 65 Men: men with risk factors for osteoporosis (50-70); all men over age 70
Ultrasound (abdominal aortic aneurysm)	Men between ages 65-75
Testing for sexually transmitted disease	Both partners should get tested prior to intercourse Any change in partners or intercourse outside partnership dictates retesting
Mental health screens	As indicated or recommended by your primary care provider
Cancer screens	See Cancer Screening Recommendations on page 185
Immunizations	See Adult Immunization Schedule on page 186

Cancer Screening Recommendations[64]

Site	Screening Recommendations
Breast	Mammogram every 1 to 2 yr in women ages 50-75
Cervix	Pap smear every 3 years until age 65 in all women with a cervix.
Colon	High-sensitivity fecal occult blood (FOBT) yearly (50-75), sigmoidoscopy every 5 yr or colonoscopy every 10 yr in all individuals ages 50-75
Lung	Low-dose computed tomography in 55- to 80-year-olds with a 30-pack-year history and who smoke or have quit in past 15 years
Oral	Evidence insufficient to recommend routine screening
Ovarian	Routine screening is not recommended
Prostate	PSA-based screening is not recommended.
Skin	Skin exams recommended by American Cancer Society
Testicular	No routine screens recommended.

IMMUNIZATIONS

Recommended Adult Immunization Schedule by Vaccine and Age Group, United States — 2015[18]

VACCINE ▼ AGE GROUP ▶	19-21 years	22-26 years	27-49 years	50-59 years	60-64 years	≥ 65 years
Influenza*,†	1 dose annually					
Tetanus, diphtheria, pertussis (Td/Tdap)*	Substitute 1-time dose of Tdap for Td booster; then boost with Td every 10 yrs					
Varicella*	2 doses					
Human papillomavirus (HPV) Female*	3 doses					
Human papillomavirus (HPV) Male*	3 doses					
Zoster						1 dose
Measles, mumps, rubella (MMR)*	1 or 2 doses					
Pneumococcal 13-valent conjugate (PCV13)*						1-time dose
Pneumococcal polysaccharide (PPSV23)			1 or 2 doses			1 dose
Meningococcal*	1 or more doses					
Hepatitis A*,†	2 doses					
Hepatitis B*	3 doses					
Haemophilus influenzae type b (Hib)*	1 or 3 doses					

*Covered by the Vaccine Injury Compensation Program

[ ] For all persons in this category who meet the age requirements and who lack documentation of vaccination or have no evidence of previous infection; zoster vaccine recommended regardless of prior episode of zoster

[ ] Recommended if some other risk factor is present (e.g., on the basis of medical, occupational, lifestyle, or other indication)

[ ] No recommendation

For complete schedule with footnotes, see: www.cdc.gov/vaccines/schedules/hcp/imz/adult.html

FACTS

USEFUL HEALTH CARE WEBSITES

Academy of Nutrition and Dietetics
www.eatright.org

American Cancer Society
www.cancer.org

American Diabetes Association
www.diabetes.org

American Heart Association
www.heart.org

American Lung Association
www.lung.org

Centers for Disease Control and Prevention
www.cdc.gov

Health.gov
www.health.gov

Healthy People
www.healthypeople.gov

Mental Health America
www.nmha.org

National Center for Complementary and Integrative Health
https://nccih.nih.gov

National Institutes of Health
health.nih.gov

U.S. Department of Health and Human Services
www.hhs.gov

WebMD
www.webmd.com

Household

Weight
    1 Tbsp = 3 tsp
    1 cup = 16 Tbsp
    1 lb = 16 oz

Volume
    1 gal = 4 qt
    1 qt = 2 pt
    1 pt = 2 cups
    1 cup = 8 oz

Metric System

Household Metric Conversions
    15 gtts = 1 mL
    1 tsp = 4-5 mL
    1 Tbsp = 15 mL
    1 cup = 240 mL
    1 pt = 480 mL
    1 qt = 960 mL
    1 gal = 3840 mL or 5 L

Weight
    1 kilogram (kg/Kg) = 1000 grams (g)
    1 gram (Gm/gm/g/G) = 1000 milligrams (mg)
    1 milligram (mg) = 1000 micrograms (mcg)

Volume
    1 liter (L) = 1000 milliliters (mL)
    1 deciliter (dL) = 100 milliliters (mL)
    1 milliliter (mL) = 1 cubic centimeter (cc)

Length
    1 meter (m) = 100 centimeters (cm)
    1 meter (m) = 1000 millimeters (mm)
    1 centimeter (cm) = 10 millimeters (mm)

■HEIGHT AND WEIGHT CONVERSION■

Height 1 in = 2.54 cm; 1 cm = 0.3937 in

in	cm	cm	in
1	2.5	1	0.4
2	5.1	2	0.8
4	10.2	3	1.2
6	15.2	4	1.6
8	20.3	5	2.0
10	25.4	6	2.4
20	50.8	8	3.1
30	76.2	10	3.9
40	101.6	20	7.9
50	127.0	30	11.8
60	152.4	40	15.7
70	177.8	50	19.7
80	203.2	60	23.6
90	227.6	70	27.6
100	254.0	80	31.5
150	381.0	90	35.4
200	508.0	100	39.4

Weight 1 lb = 0.454 kg; 1 kg = 2.204 lb

lb	kg	kg	lb
1	0.5	1	2.2
2	0.9	2	4.4
4	1.8	3	6.6
6	2.7	4	8.8
8	3.6	5	11.0
10	4.5	6	13.2
20	9.1	8	17.6
30	13.6	10	22
40	18.1	20	44
50	22.7	30	66
60	27.2	40	88
70	31.8	50	110
80	36.3	60	132
90	40.9	70	154
100	45.4	80	176
150	68.0	90	198
200	90.7	100	220

Abbreviations

Ab	abortions		**BCLS**	basic cardiac life support
abd	abdominal/abdomen		**BE**	barium enema
ABG	arterial blood gas		**bid, BID**	twice per day
ABO	three basic blood groups		**BK**	below the knee
ABO-Rh	ABO and Rh blood factors		**BM**	bowel movement
ac	before meals		**BMI**	body mass index
ACLS	advanced cardiac life support		**BMR**	basal metabolic rate
ad lib	as desired		**BOWI**	bag of waters intact
ADD	attention de cit disorder		**BP**	blood pressure, buccopulpal
ADH	antidiuretic hormone		**bpm**	beats per minute
ADL	activities of daily living		**BSA**	body surface area
AFB	acid-fast bacillus		**BSE**	breast self-examination
AFE	amniotic uid embolism		**BTL**	bilateral tubal ligation
AICD	automatic implantable cardiac de brillator		**BUN**	blood urea nitrogen
AIDS	acquired immunode ciency syndrome		**Bx**	biopsy
AK	above the knee		**c̄**	with
ALS	advanced life support, amyotrophic lateral sclerosis		**C&S**	culture and sensitivity
ALT	alanine aminotransferase		**c/o**	complains of
AM	morning		**Ca**	calcium
AMA	against medical advice		**CABG**	coronary artery bypass graft
AMI	acute myocardial infarction		**CAD**	coronary artery disease
amp	ampule		**caps**	capsule
A-P, AP, A/P	anterior-posterior		**CAT**	computerized (axial) tomography
AROM	arti cial rupture of membranes		**CBC, cbc**	complete blood cell
ASD	atrial septal defect		**CC**	chief complaint
ASHD	arteriosclerotic heart disease		**CCU**	coronary care unit, critical care unit
AST	aspartate aminotransferase		**CF**	cystic brosis
A-V, AV, A/V	arteriovenous, atrioventricular		**CHD**	congenital heart disease, coronary heart disease
			CHF	congestive heart failure
Ba	barium		**CHO**	carbohydrate
BBB	blood-brain barrier; bundle-branch block		**CK**	creatinine kinase
			cm	centimeter
			CMV	cytomegalovirus
			CNS	central nervous system
			CO	carbon monoxide; cardiac output; castor oil

CO₂	carbon dioxide	**Dx**	diagnosis
COLD	chronic obstructive lung disease		
COPD	chronic obstructive pulmonary disease	**EBV**	Epstein-Barr virus
		ECF	extended care facility, extracellular fluid
CP	cerebral palsy, cleft palate	**ECG**	electrocardiogram, electrocardiograph
CPK	creatine phosphokinase	**ECHO**	echocardiography
CPR	cardiopulmonary resuscitation	**ECT**	electroconvulsive therapy
CSF	cerebrospinal fluid; colony-stimulating factor	**ED**	emergency department
		EDB	estimated date of birth
CST	contraction stress test	**EDC**	expected date of confinement
CT	computed tomography		
CVA	cerebrovascular accident, costovertebral angle	**EDD**	estimated date of delivery
		EEG	electroencephalogram
		EENT	eye, ear, nose, throat
CVP	central venous pressure	**eff**	effacement
CXR	chest x-ray	**EFM**	electronic fetal monitor/ing
		ELISA	enzyme-linked immunosorbent assay
d	day		
D&C	dilatation and curettage	**elix**	elixir
D₅W	dextrose 5% in water	**EMG**	electromyogram
DIC	disseminated intravascular coagulation	**EMS**	emergency medical services
diff	differential blood count	**EMT**	emergency medical technician
dil	dilute, dissolve		
DKA	diabetic ketoacidosis	**epid**	epidural
dl, dL	deciliter	**epic**	episiotomy
DM	diabetes mellitus	**ER**	emergency room (hospital)
DNA	deoxyribonucleic acid	**ERV**	expiratory reserve volume
DNR	do not resuscitate	**ESR**	erythrocyte sedimentation rate
DOA	dead on arrival		
DOB	date of birth	**ESRD**	end-stage renal disease
DOE	dyspneic on exertion	**ext**	extract
DPT	diphtheria-pertussis-tetanus		
		FBS	fasting blood sugar
dr	dram	**Fe**	iron
DRG	diagnosis-related group	**FEV**	forced expiratory volume
DSM-IV	*Diagnostic and Statistical Manual of Mental Disorders*	**FH, Fhx**	family history
		FHR	fetal heart rate
		FHT	fetal heart tone
DT	delirium tremens	**fld, Fl**	fluid
DTR	deep tendon reflex		

FTT	failure to thrive
FUO	fever of unknown origin
fx	fracture
g, Gm, gm	gram
G, Gr, Grav	gravida
gal	gallon
GB	gallbladder
GC	gonococcus or gonorrheal
GDM	gestational diabetes mellitus
gest	gestation
GI	gastrointestinal
gm	gram
gr	grain
GSW	gunshot wound
gtt	drops
GU	genitourinary
Gyn	gynecology
H&P	history and physical
h, hr	hour
h/o	history of
H_2O_2	hydrogen peroxide
HAV	hepatitis A virus
Hb, Hgb	hemoglobin
HBV	hepatitis B virus
HCG	human chorionic gonadotropin
HCT	hematocrit
HDL	high-density lipoprotein
HEENT	head, eye, ear, nose, and throat
HELLP	Hemolysis, Elevated Liver enzymes, Lowered Platelets
Hg	mercury
HIV	human immunodeficiency (AIDS) virus
HPI	history of present illness
HR	heart rate
HSV	herpes simplex virus
HT, HTN	hypertension
hx, Hx	history

hypo	hypodermic
I&O	intake and output
IBW	ideal body weight
ICP	intracranial pressure
ICU	intensive care unit
ID	intradermal
IDDM	insulin-dependent diabetes mellitus
IDM	infant of a diabetic mother
IFM	internal fetal monitoring
Ig	immunoglobulin
IM	intramuscular
in	inch
IPPB	intermittent positive pressure breathing
IRV	inspiratory reserve volume
IUD	intrauterine device
IUPC	intrauterine pressure catheter
IV	intravenous
IVP	intravenous pyelogram, intravenous push
IVPB	intravenous piggyback
K^+	potassium
kg	kilogram
KCl	potassium chloride
KUB	kidney/ureter/bladder
KVO	keep vein open
L	left, liter, length, lumbar, lethal
L&D	labor and delivery
L&W	living and well
lab	laboratory
lb	pound
LDL	low-density lipoprotein
LE	lower extremity, lupus erythematosus
LGA	large for gestational age
LLE	left lower extremity
LLL	left lower lobe

LLQ	left lower quadrant
LMP	last menstrual period
LOC	level/loss of consciousness
LP	lumbar puncture
LR	lactated Ringer's
LUE	left upper extremity
LUL	left upper lobe
LUQ	left upper quadrant
LV	left ventricle
LVH	left ventricular hypertrophy
m	meter; minim
Mg	magnesium sulfate
MAP	mean arterial pressure
mcg	microgram
MCH	mean corpuscular hemoglobin
MCHC	mean corpuscular hemoglobin concentration
MCV	mean corpuscular volume, molluscum contagiosum virus
MD	muscular dystrophy
mEq	milliequivalent
MFM	Maternal-Fetal Medicine
mg	milligram
MI	myocardial infarction
ml, mL	milliliter
MLE	median episiotomy
mm	millimeter
mm Hg	millimeters of mercury
MMR	maternal mortality rate, measles-mumps-rubella
MRI	magnetic resonance imaging
MS	multiple sclerosis
MSF	meconium-stained fluid
Multip	multipara
MVA	motor vehicle accident

MVU	Montevideo unit
N&V, N/V	nausea and vomiting
npo, NPO	nothing by mouth
N/A	not applicable
Na^+	sodium
NaCl	sodium chloride
NANDA	North American Nursing Diagnosis Association
NG	nasogastric
NIBP	noninvasive blood pressure
NICU	neonatal intensive care unit
NIDDM	non–insulin-dependent diabetes mellitus
NKA	no known allergies
NS	normal saline
NST	nonstress test
O_2	oxygen
OB	obstetrics
OBS	organic brain syndrome
OOB	out of bed
OR	operating room
OT	occupational therapy
OTC	over-the-counter
oz	ounce
P	para or pulse
P-A, PA, P/A	posterior-anterior
PALS	pediatric advanced life support
Para I, II, etc	unipara, bipara, tripara, etc.
p	after
PAT	paroxysmal atrial tachycardia
pc	after meals
PCA	patient-controlled analgesia

PCWP .... pulmonary capillary wedge pressure	q3h .... every 3 hours
PDA .... patent ductus arteriosus	q4h .... every 4 hours
PE .... physical examination	qh .... every hour
PEEP .... positive end-expiratory pressure	qid, QID .... four times a day
PEFR ..peak expiratory flow rate	qs .... as sufficient
per .... through or by	qt .... quart
Peri care .... perineal care	
PERRLA ......pupils equal, round, and reactive to light and accommodation	R ...respiration, right, Rickettsia, roentgen
	R/ .... take
	R/O .... rule out
PID .... pelvic inflammatory disease	R/T .... related to
	RBC, rbc .... red blood cell
PIH............... pregnancy-induced hypertension	RDA .... recommended daily/dietary allowance
Pit ....Pitocin	RDS .... respiratory distress syndrome
PKU .... phenylketonuria	
PM .... evening	Rh ....symbol of rhesus factor, symbol for rhodium
PMH .... past medical history	
PMI .... point of maximal impulse	RLE ....right lower extremity
PMN .... polymorphonuclear neutrophil leukocytes (polys)	RLL .... right lower lobe
	RLQ .... right lower quadrant
PMS ..... premenstrual syndrome	RML ....right middle lobe of lung
PND .... paroxysmal nocturnal dyspnea	RNA .... ribonucleic acid
	ROM ....range of motion, rupture of membranes
PO, po .... orally	
PP .... postpartum	ROS .... review of systems
PPD ....purified protein derivative (TB test)	RR........................recovery room, respiratory rate
	RT .....radiation therapy, reading test, respiratory therapy
pres .... presentation	
primip .... primipara	RUE ....right upper extremity
PRN, prn .... as required	RUL .... right upper lobe
pro time .... prothrombin time	RUQ .... right upper quadrant
PSA ... prostate-specific antigen	
pt .... pint	s̄ .... without
PT .... prothrombin time, physical therapy	s/s .... signs and symptoms
	S-A, SA, S/A .... sinoatrial
PTL .... preterm labor	SCN .... special care nursery
PTT .... partial thromboplastin time	Sed rate ...... sedimentation rate
	SGA ......small for gestational age
PVC .... premature ventricular contraction	SGPT ....serum glutamic pyruvic transaminase
q .... every	SI ....Système International
q2h .... every 2 hours	

194

SIDS	sudden infant death syndrome	TPN	total parenteral nutrition
SL	sublingual	TPR	temperature, pulse, and respiration
SLE	systemic lupus erythematosus	tr, tinct	tincture
SNF	skilled nursing facility	TSE	testicular self-examination
SOB	shortness of breath	TSH	thyroid-stimulating hormone
sol	solution		
SGOT	serum glutamic oxaloacetic transaminase	tsp	teaspoon
		TURP	transurethral resection of prostate
SROM	spontaneous rupture of membranes	Tx	treatment
sta	station	UA	urinalysis
Staph	staphylococcus	UE	upper extremity
stat	immediately	ung	ointment
STD	sexually transmitted disease, skin test dose	URI	upper respiratory infection
		US	ultrasound
Strep	streptococcus	UTI	urinary tract infection
supp	suppository	VBAC	vaginal birth after cesarean
susp	suspension		
SVE	sterile vaginal examination	VC	vital capacity
		vit	vitamin
Sx	symptoms	vol	volume
syr	syrup	VS, vs	vital signs
		VSD	ventricular septal defect
T, Tbsp	tablespoon	WBC, wbc	white blood cell
T&A	tonsillectomy and adenoidectomy	WD	well developed
		WN	well nourished
tab	tablet	WNL	within normal limits
TAb	therapeutic abortion	wt	weight
TB	tuberculin, tuberculosis, tubercle bacillus		
TENS	transcutaneous electrical nerve stimulation		
TIA	transient ischemic attack		
TIBC	total iron-binding capacity		
tid, TID	three times a day		
TKO	to keep open		
TL	tubal ligation		
TM	tympanic membrane		
TMJ	temporomandibular joint		
TNTC	too numerous to count		

Error-Prone Abbreviations[33]

ABBREVIATIONS	INTENDED MEANING	MISINTERPRETATION	CORRECTION
μg	Microgram	Mistaken as "mg"	Use "mcg"
AD, AS, AU	Right ear, left ear, each ear	Mistaken as "OD," "OS," "OU" (right eye, left eye, each eye)	Use "right ear," "left ear," or "each ear"
OD, OS, OU	Right eye, left eye, each eye	Mistaken as "AD," "AS," "AU" (right ear, left ear, each ear)	Use "right eye," "left eye," or "each eye"
BT	Bedtime	Mistaken as "BID" (twice daily)	Use "bedtime"
cc	Cubic centimeters	Mistaken as "u" (units)	Use "mL"
D/C	Discharge or discontinue	Premature discontinuation of medications if D/C (intended to mean "discharge") has been misinterpreted as "discontinued" when followed by a list of discharge medications	Use "discharge" and "discontinue"
IJ	Injection	Mistaken as "IV" or "intrajugular"	Use "injection"
IN	Intranasal	Mistaken as "IM" or "IV"	Use "intranasal" or "NAS"
HS	Half-strength	Mistaken as "bedtime"	Use "half-strength" or "bedtime"
hs	At bedtime, hours of sleep	Mistaken as "half-strength"	Use "half-strength" or "bedtime"
IU	International unit	Mistaken as "IV" (intravenous) or "10" (ten)	Use "units"
o.d. or OD	Once daily	Mistaken as "right eye" (OD, oculus dexter), leading to oral liquid medications administered in the eye	Use "daily"
OJ	Orange juice	Mistaken as "OD" or "OS" (right or left eye); drugs meant to be diluted in orange juice may be given in the eye	Use "orange juice"
Per os	By mouth, orally	The "os" can be mistaken as "left eye" (OS, oculus sinister)	Use "PO," "by mouth," or "orally"
q.d. or QD	Every day	Mistaken as "q.i.d.," especially if period after the "q" or	Use "daily"

Abbreviation	Intended Meaning	Misinterpretation	Correction
	At bedtime	Mistaken as "qhr" or "every hour"	Use "at bedtime"
qn	Nightly	Mistaken as "qh" (every hour)	Use "nightly"
q.o.d. or QOD	Every other day	Mistaken as "q.d." (daily) or "q.i.d." (four times daily) if the "o" is poorly written	Use "every other day"
q1d	Daily	Mistaken as "q.i.d." (four times daily)	Use "daily"
q6PM, etc.	Every evening at 6 PM	Mistaken as "every 6 hours"	Use "6 PM nightly" or "6 PM daily"
SC, SQ, sub q	Subcutaneous	SC mistaken as "SL" (sublingual); SQ mistaken as "5 every;" the "q" in "sub q" has been mistaken as "every" (e.g., a heparin dose ordered "sub q 2 hours before surgery" misunderstood as every 2 hours before surgery)	Use "subcut" or "subcutaneously"
ss	Sliding scale (insulin) or ½ (apothecary)	Mistaken as "55"	Spell out "sliding scale;" Use "one-half" or "½"
SSRI	Sliding scale regular insulin	Mistaken as "selective-serotonin reuptake inhibitor"	Spell out "sliding scale (insulin)"
SSI	Sliding scale insulin	Mistaken as "Strong Solution of Iodine" (Lugol's)	Spell out "sliding scale (insulin)"
i/d	One daily	Mistaken as "tid"	Use "1 daily"
TIW or tiw	3 times a week	Mistaken as "3 times a day" or "twice in a week"	Use "3 times weekly"
U or u	Unit	Mistaken as the number 0 or 4, causing a 10-fold overdose or greater (e.g., 4U seen as "40" or 4u seen as "44"); mistaken as "cc" so dose given in volume instead of units (e.g., 4u seen as "4cc")	Use "unit"
UD	As directed ("ut dictum")	Mistaken as "unit dose" (e.g., diltiazem 125 mg IV infusion "UD" misinterpreted as meaning to give the entire infusion as a unit (bolus) dose)	Use "as directed"

Error-Prone Designations[33]

DOSE DESIGNATIONS AND OTHER INFORMATION	INTENDED MEANING	MISINTERPRETATION	CORRECTION
Trailing zero after decimal point (e.g. 1.0 mg)	1 mg	Mistaken as 10 mg if the decimal point is not seen	Do not use trailing zeros for doses expressed in whole numbers
"Naked" decimal point (e.g., .5 mg)	0.5 mg	Mistaken as 5 mg if the decimal point is not seen	Use zero before a decimal point when the dose is less than a whole unit
Drug name and dose run together (especially problematic for drug names that end in "l" such as Inderal40 mg; Tegretol300 mg)	Inderal 40 mg Tegretol 300 mg	Mistaken as Inderal 140 mg Mistaken as Tegretol 1300 mg	Place adequate space between the drug name, dose, and unit of measure
Numerical dose and unit of measure run together (e.g., 10mg, 100mL)	10 mg 100 mL	The "m" is sometimes mistaken as a zero or two zeros, risking a 10- to 100-fold overdose	Place adequate space between the dose and unit of measure
Abbreviations such as mg. or mL. with a period following the abbreviation	mg mL	The period is unnecessary and could be mistaken as the number 1 if written poorly	Use mg, mL, etc., without a terminal period
Large doses without properly placed commas (e.g. 100000 units; 1000000 units)	100,000 units 1,000,000 units	100000 has been mistaken as 10,000 or 1,000,000; 1000000 has been mistaken as 100,000	Use commas for dosing units at or above 1,000, or use words such as 100 "thousand" or 1 "million" to improve readability

Patient Safety Systems: Building Blocks[36]

Improvement Engine

RPI
- Lean, six sigma and change management
- Investments in training
- Proactive approaches prevail
- Transparency in data use
- Celebrate improvements

The Glue

Safety Culture
- Patient centered, safety first
- Voicing concerns
- Robust reporting
- Address behaviors that undermine safety culture
- Engagement in learning and improvement
- Values are hard wired into recruitment and on boarding process

The Foundation

Leadership
- Safety is #1 priority
- Models a culture of safety
- Commitment demonstrated by resources
- Values transparency
- Learning organization
- Maintains full accountability
- Data driven

SOURCES

1. Aehlert B: *ACLS study guide,* ed 4, St Louis, 2012 Mosby.

2. Aehlert B: *ECGs made easy,* ed 5, St Louis, 2015, Mosby.

3. Aehlert B: *Mosby's comprehensive pediatric emergency care,* St Louis, 2007, Mosby.

4. Aehlert B: *Rapid ACLS,* ed 2 revised reprint, St Louis, 2012, Mosby.

5. AHI of Indiana, Inc. All rights reserved. US Patent No. 7,282,031 and No. 7,682,308. Reproduction and use prohibited except by written permission from AHI of Indiana, Inc.

6. American Association of Blood Banks: *Standards for blood banks and transfusion services.* ed 29, Bethesda, 2014, The Association.

7. American College of Obstetricians and Gynecologists (ACOG): Executive summary: Hypertension in pregnancy. *Obstet Gynecol* 122, 1122-1131, 2013.

8. American Geriatrics Society 2012 Beers Criteria Update Expert Panel: American Geriatrics Society updated Beers criteria for potentially inappropriate medication use in older adults. *J Am Geriatr Soc* 60:616-631, 2012.

9. American Heart Association: *ACLS provider manual,* 2011, American Heart Association.

10. American Heart Association: 2010 *Handbook of emergency cardiovascular care for healthcare providers,* 2010, American Heart Association.

11. The American Heart Association 2010 Guidelines for Cardiopulmonary Resuscitation and Emergency Cardiovascular Care, *Circulation* 122 (suppl 3): S639-S946, 2010.

12. Barkin R, Rosen P: *Emergency pediatrics: a guide to ambulatory care,* ed 6, St Louis, 2004, Mosby.

13. Betz CL, Sowden LA: *Mosby's pediatric nursing reference,* ed 6, St Louis, Mosby, 2008.

14. Brooke P, Bullock R: Validation of a 6-item cognitive impairment test with a view to primary care, *Int J Geriatr Psychiatry* 14:936-940, 1999.

5. Brown JB, et al: Development of the Woman Abuse Screening Tool for use in family practice. *Fam Med* 28:422-428, 1996.

6. California Department of Public Health, *Network for a Healthy California*. Adapted from The Activity Pyramid. Pyramids of Health, Park Nicollet Health Source 2002. www.network-toolbox.cdph.ca.gov/en/pdf/Handouts/Hand PAPyramid.pdf, 2002 (Accessed May 13, 2015.)

7. Center for Drug Evaluation and Research: *Name Differentiation Project, Rockville, MD, 2002, Center for Drug Evaluation and Research.* www.fda.gov/drugs/ drugsafety/medicationerrors/, 2002 (Accessed April 10, 2015.)

8. Centers for Disease Control: *Recommended Adult Immunization Schedule-United States, 2015.* www.cdc.gov/vaccines/schedules/, 2015 (Accessed May 15, 2015.)

9. Centers for Disease Control: *Recommended Childhood and Adolescent Immunization Schedule-United States, 2015.* www.cdc.gov/vaccines/schedules/, 2015 (Accessed May 7, 2015.)

10. Centers for Disease Control: *Recommended immunizations for pregnant women 2015.* www.cdc.gov/vaccines/, 2015 (Accessed April 23, 2015.)

1. Chernecky CC, et al: *Saunders nursing survival guide: fluids and electrolytes,* ed 2, Philadelphia, 2006, Saunders.

2. Clayton B, Willihnganz M: *Basic pharmacology for nurses,* ed 16, St Louis, 2013, Mosby.

3. Corning B: *Mosby's PDQ for respiratory care,* St Louis, 2013, Mosby.

4. Edelman M: *Health promotion throughout the life span,* ed 8, St Louis, 2013, Mosby.

5. ENA: *Sheehy's Manual of emergency care,* ed 7, St Louis, 2013, Mosby.

6. Engel JK: *Mosby's pocket guide to pediatric assessment,* ed 5, St Louis, 2006, Mosby.

7. Fultz J, Stuart P: *Mosby's emergency nursing reference,* ed 3, St Louis, 2005, Mosby.

28. Gahart BL, Nazareno AR: *2015 Intravenous medications,* ed 31, St Louis, 2015, Mosby.

29. Harkreader H, Hogan MA: *Fundamentals of nursing: caring and clinical judgment,* ed 3, St Louis, 2007, Mosby.

30. Hockenberry MJ, Wilson D: *Wong's essentials of pediatric nursing,* ed 9, St Louis, 2013, Mosby.

31. Hockenberry MJ, Wilson D: *Wong's nursing care of infants and children,* ed 9, St Louis, 2011, Mosby.

32. Hockenberry MJ, Wilson D: *Wong's nursing care of infants and children,* ed 10, St Louis, 2015, Mosby.

33. Institute for Safe Medication Practices: *ISMP list of error-prone abbreviations, symbols, and dose designations.* www.ismp.org, 2015 (Accessed May 18, 2015.)

34. James PA, et al: 2014 Evidence Based Guideline for the Management of High Blood Pressure in Adults: Report from the Panel Appointed to the Eight Joint National Committee (JNC 8), *JAMA* 311:507-520, 2014.

35. Jarvis C: *Physical examination and health assessment,* ed 6, St Louis, 2012, Saunders.

36. Joint Commission International. *Joint Commission Enterprise Leaders Engage in Crucial Health Care Conversations in the People's Republic of China and South Korea.* http://www .jointcommissioninternational.org, 2015 (Accessed May 13, 2015.)

37. Kee JL, et al: *Pharmacology: a patient-centered nursing process approach,* ed 8, St Louis, 2014, Saunders.

38. Kizior RJ, Hodgson BB: *Saunders nursing drug handbook 2015,* Philadelphia, 2015, Saunders.

39. Leasia MS, Monahan FD: *A practical guide to health assessment,* ed 2, Philadelphia, 2002, WB Saunders.

40. Lewis SM, et al: *Medical-surgical nursing: assessment and management of clinical problems,* ed 9, St Louis, 2014, Mosby.

41. Linton A, Maebius N: *Introduction to medical-surgical nursing,* ed 4, St Louis, 2007, Saunders.

2. Lowdermilk DL, et al: *Maternity & women's health care,* ed 11, St Louis, 2016, Mosby.

3. Lowdermilk DL, Perry SE: *Maternity nursing,* ed 8, revised reprint, St Louis, 2014, Mosby.

4. Massachusetts Nurses Association (MNA): *Nurses' six rights for safe medication administration,* Developed by the Congress on Nursing Practice; Canton, MA. 2006 and included in a MNA Position Statement on Medication Error. Available at: www.massnurses.org/nurse_practice/sixrights.htm.

5. Meiner SE: *Gerontologic nursing,* ed 5, St. Louis 2015, Mosby.

6. Miller LA, et al: *Pocket guide to fetal monitoring and assessment,* ed 7, St Louis, 2013, Mosby.

7. National Heart, Lung, and Blood Institute, National Institutes of Health: *Classification of overweight and obesity by BMI, waist circumference, and associated disease risks.* http://www.nhlbi.nih.gov/health/educational/lose_wt/BMI/bmi_dis.htm.

8. National Institute on Alcohol Abuse and Alcoholism (NIAAA): *Helping patients who drink too much: a clinician's guide, Patient Education Materials: What's a standard drink.* HYPERLINK "http://www.niaaa.nih.gov" www.niaaa.nih.gov, 2005. (Accessed September 7, 2011.)

9. Norton D, et al: *An investigation of geriatric nursing problems in the hospital.* London, 1962, National Corporation for the Care of Old People (now the Centre for Policy on Ageing). Reprinted with permission.

0. Pagana KD, Pagana TJ: *Mosby's manual of diagnostic and laboratory tests,* ed 5, St Louis, 2014, Mosby.

1. Perry AG, Potter PA: *Mosby's pocket guide to basic skills and procedures,* ed 8, St Louis, 2014, Mosby.

2. Perry AG, Potter PA. *Clinical nursing skills & techniques,* ed 8, St Louis, 2014, Mosby.

3. Peterson V: *Clinical companion for fundamentals of nursing: Just the facts,* ed 8, St Louis, 2013, Mosby.

4. Potter PA, Perry AG: *Fundamentals of nursing,* ed 8, St Louis, 2013, Mosby.

5. Seidel HM, et al: *Seidel's guide to physical examination,* ed 8, St Louis, 2015, Mosby.

56. Siegal JD, et al: *Guidelines for isolation precautions: preventing transmission of infectious agents in healthcare settings,* 2007 (Accessed March 15, 2015.)

57. Skidmore-Roth L: *Mosby's 2015 nursing drug reference,* ed 24, St Louis, 2015, Mosby.

58. Spong CY: Defining "Term" pregnancy: Recommendations from the defining pregnancy workgroup, *JAMA,* 309(23):2445-2446, 2013.

59. Stillwell S: *Mosby's critical care nursing reference,* ed 4, St Louis, 2006, Mosby.

60. Touhy TA, Jett KF: *Ebersole and Hess Gerontological nursing & healthy aging,* ed 4, St Louis, 2014, Mosby.

61. Trelease CC: Developing standards for wound care *Ostomy Wound Manage,* 26:50, 1988. Used with permission.

62. US Department of Health and Human Services: *2008 Physical Activity Guidelines for Americans.* www.health.gov/PAGuidelines/pdf/paguide.pdf, 2008 (Accessed May 13, 2015.)

63. US Department of Health and Human Services, National Institutes of Health, US National Library of Medicine, Bethesda, MD. *Health Screening, 2015.* www.nlm.nih.gov/medlineplus/healthscreening.html (Accessed May 15, 2015.)

64. US Preventive Services Taskforce: *Guide to clinical preventive services, 2014.* www.ahrq.gov/professionals/clinicians-providers/guidelines-recommendations/guide/, 2014. (Accessed May 15, 2015.)

65. Wilson S, Giddens J: *Health Assessment for nursing practice,* ed 5, St Louis, 2013, Mosby.

66. Wold G: *Basic geriatric nursing,* ed 5, St Louis, 2012, Mosby.

67. Wolf R: Risk assessment instruments, *National Center on Elder Abuse Newsletter*, 3(1) 2000. Reprinted courtesy of National Center on Elder Abuse.

68. World Health Organization: *WHO guidelines on hand hygiene in health care.* http://whqlibdoc.who.int/publications/2009 (Accessed March 15, 2015.)

INDEX

MOSBY'S
PDQ *for* RN
Practical, Detailed, Quick

4e

The perfect rapid reference for the clinical setting!

When in doubt, check this handy guide to important facts, formulas, and procedures used in the clinical setting. It offers quick access to details you need but don't usually memorize, such as signs and symptoms, medications, conversions, abbreviations, and normal/abnormal ranges for laboratory tests.

OUTSTANDING FEATURES:

NEW clinical developments, including screening guidelines and drug information

NEW assessment tools for pain, nutrition, and alcohol abuse

NEW! Expanded topics such as oxygen delivery, hypoglycemic drugs, and cardiac rhythms

10 tabbed, color-coded sections for easier lookup

Colorful charts and tables summarizing key data

Durable pages can withstand the wear
and tear of daily use on the job!

ISBN 978-0-323-40028-2

9 780323 400282

ELSEVIER
elsevier.com